MW01166353

AIDS: The Drug and Alcohol Connection

What Health Care Professionals Need To Know

Larry Siegel, M.D., and Milan Korcok

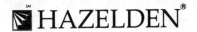

HAZELDEN®

First published June 1989

ISBN: 0-89486-573-0

Library of Congress Catalog Card Number: 89-80218

Printed in the United States of America

Editor's Note:

Hazelden Educational Materials offers a variety of information
on chemical dependency and related areas. Our publications do
not necessarily represent Hazelden or its programs, nor do they
officially speak for any Twelve Step organization.

With gratitude and love to Dana Finnegan for helping create this opportunity; to the late Dr. Tom Smith for his inspiration; to Dr. John Jonikas for being there; and to Reba Siegel Schwager for putting me on the planet.

—Dr. Larry Siegel

Contents

CHAPTER ONE

Understanding AIDS

Do you have a clear understanding of AIDS — the Acquired Immune Deficiency Syndrome? Do you know what it is? Do you know how it travels? Do you know why it has spread so quickly among drug users? Do you know what you can do to protect yourself and others? We hope this book will help you answer yes to these questions. All people need to be able to answer yes because AIDS is one the most serious public health problems being faced by this generation.

In the brochure, *Understanding AIDS*, sent to all American homes in 1988 by the U.S. Public Health Service, Surgeon General C. Everett Koop, declared: "Stopping AIDS is up to you, your family, and your loved ones."

He went on to say that talking about AIDS issues may not be easy. "But now you must discuss them....We must all get to know about AIDS....Get involved."

Dr. Koop's appeals were meant to encourage education of all people of all ages, including youngsters in the early grades of school. No one can afford not to know about AIDS.

The Special Role of Chemical Dependency Caregivers

Some groups, especially those already in the front-line fight against this disease, need to have AIDS information brought into their daily working lives. They need it because they have an opportunity to do something about it, to reduce its destruction, and to prevent its occurrence in people they deal with every day.

Among health care providers, those who work with chemically dependent persons have a unique opportunity to provide education about AIDS and to help change the high-risk behaviors that the Human Immunodeficiency Virus (HIV) thrives on.

It is our purpose in this book to offer a clear view of the connection between AIDS and mood-altering drugs — including alcohol — and to discuss what health care professionals can and should do about it.

We will cite information about the transmission of the AIDS virus, the people it's affecting most acutely, the educational and preventive efforts being used to contain the spread, and the advances being made to prolong life among those with AIDS and related diseases.

Much of the data we report will be a distillation of various studies and will already have become part of the mainstream knowledge about AIDS. In those cases, we will not cite all of the scientific sources, but we will refer you to relevant books and articles that cover and expand on the points being made. Occasionally, when we feel an individual report reveals new or especially provocative information not yet widely known, we'll cite the specific source. Citations won't always be possible, however, because some of what we report will have been gleaned from papers and lectures not yet published, from informal discussions between scientists and clinicians, and from seminars and meetings where experts have freely exchanged views and traded observations and hypotheses.

We'll attempt to clearly differentiate between what has been established scientifically and what is still in the preliminary observation and hypothetical stage.

We'll also present patient case histories from our medical files to give the clinical points we make a human dimension. To avoid unnecessary repetition, we will occasionally consolidate clinical findings from more than one patient into a composite example. But where we do this you can be assured that the composite findings reflect real people in real situations. In all cases, actual names have been changed.

Much of the data about the spread of AIDS, the numbers involved, and the populations most affected derive from the continuing investigative and surveillance efforts of the Centers for Disease Control (CDC), which is a part of the U.S. Public Health Service. The CDC is the greatest single repository of information about AIDS, and it maintains day by day updates available to interested professionals, the media, and the public.

In addition to scientific journals and the CDC, we have also relied on observations and reports from meetings such as the National Forum on AIDS and Chemical Dependency organized by the American Medical Society on Alcoholism and Other Drug Dependencies (AMSAODD).

Reports of these conference proceedings (available from AMSAODD, 12 West Twenty-First Street, New York, New York, 10010, or from your medical library) have been a rich source of new, cutting-edge information about the critical role chemical dependency professionals have in curbing the spread of AIDS.

There are also several books and other reference materials that we recommend to you which we feel will enhance your knowledge about AIDS, chemical dependency, and living and recovering from the effects of AIDS. We have appended these as a general reference source (see Suggested Reading at the back of this book).

Throughout this book, we will describe experiences and we will offer hope. This book is for physicians and all other health care providers who work with individuals and families with AIDS, with people who are HIV positive and worried about their future, with persons and families at risk or already beset by problems with alcohol or other drugs, and with patients and families in need of education about how to live healthy lives.

The Special Links between AIDS and Drug Use

AIDS is a biopsychosocial disease. It is influenced by physical, psychological, behavioral, and environmental conditions. It affects the mind, the body, and the emotions — components that are interconnected with what some call the spirit. In those respects at least, AIDS is similar to alcoholism and other drug addiction. The diseases are similar in one other respect: there is no single, simple "magic bullet" to either cure them or prevent their occurrence.

A number of authorities have emphasized the widespread use of alcohol and other drugs among people who develop AIDS. And while it is well known that a high prevalence of seropositivity to HIV exists in IV drug using populations (up to 80 percent in some parts of the country),[1] there are now reports of increasing seropositivity in other chemically dependent patients.

In one large drug program that has done HIV testing, the seroprevalence was about 13 percent.[2] In another survey, 4 percent of 2,302 consecutive adult patients brought into an inner city hospital emergency department during a six week period had unrecognized HIV infection.[3]

Development of a vaccine or cure for AIDS will be slow. The presence of multiple strains of the virus, the "in vivo" mutation of the virus itself, the insertion of the virus into the basic genetic material of the cells it invades, and the apparent lack of protection of the naturally occurring antibodies, are all major impediments to vaccine development.

Chemical dependency professionals are trained to help people discover, within themselves, the strength and the discipline to change their behaviors. This is the key to avoiding risk of infection, and to retarding or preventing progression of the disease if infection has already occurred. Chemical dependency caregivers are also skilled in helping patients, families, spouses, significant others, and friends deal with the moral and social issues so much a part of the AIDS problem — just as they have been a part of alcoholism and other drug addiction.

Enormous work and public education achieved the widespread acceptance of alcoholism and other drug addiction as being a disease rather than a moral issue. For the most part, the person with AIDS has not won the same regard. But no one is better equipped to help him or her win it than the caregivers who work with alcohol and other drug abusers every day.

The treatment techniques to achieve these ends are in place. They are part of the daily repertoire of chemical dependency professionals, family physicians, internists, obstetricians and gynecologists, psychiatrists, nurses, social workers, counselors, and many mental health professionals.

In the succeeding chapters we will address all of these issues, with special emphasis on confidentiality, testing, and legal concerns. Most important, we will try to encourage a sense of respect toward clients and patients in need of help. We'll seek to ensure that professionals in a position to help, first of all do clients and patients no harm.

Some of these points and various references will be discussed in more than one chapter. In writing this book, we have purposely repeated some points to emphasize their relevance to different contexts of the interface between AIDS and chemical dependency. We intend this approach to facilitate those who read chapters according to subject interest rather than from beginning to end.

ENDNOTES

1. C. R. Schuster, "NIAAA/NIDA Research on Alcohol and Drug Abuse and AIDS — Current Projects and Future Needs," in *Keeping Hope Alive*, Milan Korcok, ed. (Providence Rhode Island: Manisses Communications 1988), 47.

2. J. M. Jacobson, et al., "Human Immunodeficiency Virus (HIV) and Hepatitis B Virus (HBV) Infection in an Alco-

holic Population," *Alcoholism, Clinical and Experimental Research*, vol. 12, no. 1 (February 1988), 192.

3. G. D. Kelen, et al., "Unrecognized Human Immunodeficiency Virus Infection In Emergency Department Patients," *New England Journal of Medicine* vol. 318, no. 25 (23 June 1988), 1,645.

CHAPTER TWO

What Is AIDS?

We are all surrounded by a variety of microorganisms that can make us ill — in the air we breathe, on our pets, in the foods we eat.

Normally, we are protected from these potential intruders by powerful barriers, the most important being our skin and the mucous membrane linings of our mouth, rectum, vagina, or penis.

But if there is a break in the skin or membrane, caused perhaps by the trauma of rectal intercourse or by needle puncture, then the organisms previously kept out can get in and begin their mischief.

If that happens, other defenses come into play. Much like a good football team, the body does not depend on a single line of defense. It has secondary defenders who come into action if the first line breaks down or is penetrated. In fact, it has defenders all the way down the field.

Most important of these defenders, especially in relationship to AIDS, are the blood's own T-helper cells.

T-Cells — The Heart of the Defense

The story of these cells, how they function, and what their role is in our complex defense system is essential to understanding how the Human Immunodeficiency Virus, normally a weak and insipid organism, can cause such havoc in some — though not all — people.

Imagine being in a doctor's office, hospital, or clinic and having a test tube of blood drawn from your arm. After the blood is drawn, it is put into a centrifuge and spun down. The bottom 45 percent of the contents is red blood cells. They contain hemoglobin that carries the oxygen necessary for survival of our tissues. The top layer, little more than half the contents, is plasma, which is mostly water.

Between the two, there is a thin line of cells called the *buffy coat layer*, which consists of white blood cells. These in turn are made of polymorphonuclear leukocytes, basophils, eosinophils, monocytes (which are called macrophages when they lodge in tissues), and several other types of cells.

The cells of most concern in relation to HIV and AIDS are lymphocytes, white blood cells that can be further divided into two groups: the T and B lymphocytes (T for the ones that originate in the thymus gland, just under the sternum or breastbone, and B for those that originate in the bone marrow.)

We can further subdivide T cells into "helper" cells (T-4) and "suppressor" (T-8) cells. The main pathophysiologic defect in a person with AIDS is the loss or impairment of T-helper cells and the subsequent reduced ratio of T-4 to T-8 or suppressor cells.

For example, if the number of T-4 cells are reduced while the number of T-8 cells remain constant or increases, then it is said that the T-4:T-8 ratio — normally one or greater — drops. That's what usually occurs in persons with AIDS.

If ordinarily nonpathogenic or dormant microorganisms invade while the T-4 cells are reduced or impaired, the invaders have an opportunity to cause infections and diseases that would normally be deflected. Thus they are called *opportunistic infections or illnesses.* AIDS is the occurrence of opportunistic infections or tumors that normally would not have had the opportunity to thrive if the body's defenders, the T-4 cells, were performing properly. Opportunistic illnesses and infections often cause the death of people with AIDS.

The process of malfunctioning T-4 cells is not a new discovery. It has been studied intently long before we knew about AIDS. All persons who receive transplanted organs — kidneys, hearts, livers — are given medication to suppress the function of T-4 cells whose job it is to help the body reject the new organ. It is, after all, an alien organ and the T-4 cell doesn't recognize it for what it is — a potential lifesaver for its host. So it attacks, and medication must be used to ward off that attack. Transplant patients who are given medication to suppress their T-4 cells (to prevent rejection of their new organs) are thus in a situation resembling patients with AIDS. The suppression of T-4 cells makes them more vulnerable to the same opportunistic infections and tumors that AIDS patients are vulnerable to. The difference is that their immune deficiency is less severe and can be controlled by altering the dosages of the immunosuppressive medications. It is also reversible if the medications are withdrawn.

Drug Use Compromises Immunity

The issue of immune suppression is particularly relevant to health care providers and patients in chemical dependency treatment because it is widely thought that one of the effects of alcoholism or addiction to other drugs is suppressed immunity.[1] If that is so, drug abusers would appear to be at increased risk for AIDS or AIDS-related infections and diseases. A more complete discussion of drug effects on immune function and on behavioral disinhibition is included in Chapter Four.

Most investigators believe that with AIDS, the T-4 cells are lost or destroyed by what has come to be known as the Human Immunodeficiency Virus. Thus, the presence of HIV in the blood tells us who is at high-risk for developing AIDS. Its presence is not, however, an assurance that the host will go on to develop AIDS.

What the HIV Test Tells Us

There are now various tests that are capable of telling us if HIV has been present in the body. If it has, then the body has generated antibodies — which form in reaction to an intruder entering the body. The Enzyme-Linked Immunosorbent Assay (ELISA) detects the presence of such antibodies and is widely used to screen persons at high risk for AIDS. The ELISA test is not infallible, however. (More about this topic will be discussed in Chapters Nine and Ten.)

The more involved Western Blot test is used to confirm the results of the ELISA test. Without such confirmation, a single positive result on an ELISA can't be used as definitive proof of the presence of HIV. There are also antigen specific tests that can detect the presence of a live infectious virus — the organism that invades the body and generates production of antibodies. But these tests are expensive and are so far confined mainly to major research centers.

The existing tests most widely used to detect the presence of HIV, such as the ELISA, really detect only the footprint of the virus. They can determine that the virus was there. They can not determine that it is still there, that it is infectious, or that the person being tested will necessarily develop AIDS. The very T-4 cells that would ordinarily fight off not only the opportunistic infections that kill people with AIDS, but the HIV virus itself become the targets of HIV. And as HIV focuses on these targets, it is often helped along its destructive course by added *cofactors* that weaken the body and make it more susceptible to infection or illness.

Cofactors and Fellow Travelers

Cofactors are circumstances or agents that contribute to the onset of some other event. To use an analogy, an alcoholic who continues to drink heavily has a higher risk of dying from mouth and throat cancers than does a nondrinker. But, adding heavy smoking to the alcoholic's daily drug intake will cause those risks to soar even higher.

In the development of AIDS, the role of cofactors is getting a lot of attention since it's apparent that more than half of those who are exposed to or infected by HIV have not gone on to develop AIDS. This simple, but crucial fact raises the possibility that by defining what these cofactors are and pro-tecting against them, HIV positive people might be able to greatly decrease their chances of progressing to AIDS.

Alcohol and other drug abuse — which suppresses parts of the immune system — might be among these cofactors. So might poor nutrition, negative mental attitudes, other ill-nesses, and high-risk behaviors such as repeated, indiscrim-inate sex.

Let's look at a specific case from our medical files. As in all subsequent case history reports in this book, all names have been changed for obvious reasons.

Case History

Russ, a twenty-six year old alcoholic gay man has been in and out of AA and treatment programs for several years. He has also had a long-term relationship with a nonalcoholic man twenty years older than himself.

Russ began to have increasing fatigue, night sweats, diarrhea, and he lost seven pounds over a month. He sought the help of his phy-sician. He was found to have thrush (an oral fungal infection often found in people who go on to AIDS), and he subsequently tested positive for HIV. His partner was HIV negative.

Russ' intense fear of his own death and of infecting his partner motivated him to stay away from alcohol. He began to attend AA meetings regularly and has done so ever since.

Two years later he remains sober and medically stable. His lover remains seronegative, and they continue to have an active sexual relationship.

For those in the alcohol and chemical dependency field, it's both critical and fulfilling to realize that by dealing with the drug use of their AIDS and HIV infected patients, they may be defeating the cofactors that represent their patients' greatest risk.

Infection in Health Care Workers

There have been thousands of documented cases of health care workers being exposed to HIV by having AIDS patients' blood or other body fluids splashed on them. But according to the continuing surveillance studies of health care workers by the Centers for Disease Control, as of November 1988, only seventeen of these workers have been infected by HIV.[2] Moreover, the CDC estimates the risk of infection by HIV after such exposure to be less than .5 percent. And most infection probably requires repeated exposure plus other susceptibility.

In fact, HIV is a very weak, puny virus and is easily killed by ordinary household detergents or diluted bleach. And while its effect can be devastating, it's important to understand that the only documented means of HIV transmission is by an infected person's blood or semen getting into someone else's body. This could include the infection of a fetus, or of a young child through the breast milk of an infected mother. (We will further discuss AIDS and children in Chapter Three.)

Studies have shown that among women with AIDS in the U.S., 52 percent have been intravenous drug users and another 21 percent have contracted AIDS through heterosexual contact, most of it with IV drug users.[3] They also show that though women represent only 8 percent of the national total of adult AIDS cases, three-quarters of these women have been involved either directly or secondarily with IV drug users.

CDC Projections

The CDC, which records all reports of AIDS on a day-to-day basis, estimates that more than 1.5 million Americans have been exposed to HIV as of 1988, and by the mid-1990s that tally may run as high as ten million. The CDC continuously publishes its data in *Morbidity and Mortality Weekly Report* and in the major scientific publications available in most libraries.

As of 28 February, 1989, 87,188 persons in the U.S. had developed full-blown AIDS. Many more suffer from lesser degrees of illness — sometimes called AIDS Related Conditions (ARC). In fact, some people with ARC or other HIV related diseases become so ill they die without ever having met the specific criteria for AIDS diagnosis established by the CDC.

While these classifications are somewhat useful, many patients develop AIDS without ever having had ARC, and most people with HIV infection have so far not become ill at all.

HIV Spectrum Disease: Signs and Symptoms

It is probably more productive to view HIV infection as the marker for disease and to call it *HIV Spectrum Disease*. There are varying degrees of HIV disease, from well to mild to moderately ill (for example, a person may experience fever, weight loss, swollen lymph glands, thrush, shingles, and mild neurocognitive defects) to life threatening (for example, pneumocystis carinii pneumonia, advanced Kaposi's Sarcoma, cryptococcal meningitis, and disseminated cytomegalovirus). In addition, certain bacterial diseases are more common in AIDS patients (tuberculosis, pneumococcal pneumonia, and salmonella gastroenteritis).

Because of the possibility of infection by this wide range of diseases and the uncertainty about who is or is not infected by HIV, the Public Health Service recommends the use of

Universal Body Substance Isolation precautions, or more simply Universal Precautions in working with all patients. (More about these precautions will be discussed in Chapter Seven.)

The average time from infection to AIDS in those who develop it is about eight years. The outer range, as it's known now, is eleven years from infection to AIDS, though mathematical projections have been made suggesting the outer range may be even longer.

There are, however, growing numbers of exceptions to these averages. And there is a need to reemphasize that HIV exposure doesn't necessarily mean infection; HIV infection doesn't necessarily mean AIDS; AIDS doesn't necessarily mean death.

As will be discussed more extensively in Chapter Three, most people infected by HIV have not developed AIDS. Different groups of people progressed to AIDS in 1981 more rapidly than others — IV drug users progressed much faster than non-IV drug using gay men, and a few people have possibly "cleared" their bodies of HIV and have become seronegative.

Survival for many years occurs and is becoming more common. There is, in fact, CDC data that shows that up to 10 percent of people diagnosed with AIDS through 1982 were still alive six years later.[4] And in some groups — such as gay men with Kaposi's sarcoma, survival can go well beyond that. (More about that in Chapters Three and Twelve.)

In summary, recognizing how difficult it is to get infected by this weak virus, and how not everyone who is infected by it dies, is an important step in allaying the personal fear of both the patient and the caregiver.

ENDNOTES

1. Larry Siegel, "AIDS Relationship to Alcohol and Other Drugs," *Journal of Substance Abuse Treatment* 3 (1986): 271.

2. R. Marcus, et al., "Surveillance of Health Care Workers Exposed to Blood from Patients Infected with the Human

Immunodeficiency Virus," *New England Journal of Medicine* vol. 319, no. 17 (27 October 1988): 1118.

3. M. Guinan and A. Hardy, "Epidemiology of AIDS in Women in the United States — 1981 through 1986," *Journal of the American Medical Association* vol. 257, no. 15 (17 April 1987): 2039.

4. Larry Siegel, "AIDS: Perceptions versus Realities," *Journal of Psychoactive Drugs* vol. 20, no. 2 (April/June 1988): 149.

CHAPTER THREE

Epidemiology

Who gets infected by HIV? Who is at risk? Who gets AIDS? These are among the key public health questions of the twentieth century.

If we look closely at *how* people get infected instead of *who* gets infected, our knowledge about the spread of AIDS becomes clearer. Certainly, no one should assume that because they are not black, gay, Hispanic, living in Africa, or because they are strict about using "clean works" for their IV drugs, that they are immune from HIV infection. Such assumptions can be dangerous.

Who Is at Risk?

No one is immune from HIV infection. But the truth is that HIV is not easy to catch. Those who do, must work at it.

The infectious agent must first get inside the body. Only then is there the opportunity for it to infect its host, and only after that is there the possibility that such infection will develop into AIDS. For that to happen, there must be an opening or a break in the skin or protective membranes in the rectum, vagina, or mouth. Only then can the infected cells from one person get into another person.

The most common ways infection happens is by vaginal or rectal sexual intercourse without condoms, or by the sharing of unsterile, unclean, drug injection equipment. It is a matter of behaviors.

Risk by Behavior

AIDS is not an illness of high-risk people, but of high-risk behaviors. And it is most prevalent in the geographic regions of the United States where high-risk behaviors such as intravenous drug use are most common — New York, California, and Florida. But this doesn't suggest AIDS is a localized threat. It isn't. It has been reported in every state and most countries of the world.

The highest risk behaviors are receptive anal intercourse without a condom, and intravenous drug injection using equipment shared with other people. Women having unprotected vaginal intercourse with infected males are also at substantial risk.

Note that we're not talking about sexuality or the relative risks of being gay or straight. Anyone in any population group can be at high or low risk. Risk depends not on who you are, but what you do. It is known, for example, that 25 percent of all American sexually active women have practiced rectal intercourse, and 10 percent do so regularly.[1] That is high-risk behavior — even when practiced by people in otherwise low-risk groups, such as women who don't use drugs.[2]

The issue is behavior, not sexuality, race, or whether you like to eat brussel sprouts!

Risk by Pregnancy and Birth

The scientific literature shows a close relationship between AIDS in children and their mother's drug abuse.

Knowledge of how HIV is transmitted to children is important to caregivers who counsel chemically dependent women after they become pregnant, and, in many cases, before they become pregnant. They can help women patients make informed decisions about pregnancy.

HIV can also be transmitted perinatally from an infected

mother to her baby while the baby is in the uterus. It is also possible that infection might occur through breast feeding. It's important, therefore, that all women considering pregnancy should seriously think about being tested for HIV before they become pregnant and should consult a physician if their test result is positive.

In such case, counseling is very important, especially if the women are drug users. Drug using pregnant women experience many obstetrical complications. They have a high rate of infection, premature labor, and a high incidence of fetal loss. Adding the possibility of HIV infection greatly increases the number of problems these women and their babies must face.

According to a report prepared for the U.S. Department of Health and Human Services by the National Institute of Child Health and Human Development, 1,291 cases of AIDS had been reported among infants and children under age thirteen between 1981 and the end of 1988. Of these, 717 had already died. Another study shows the distribution of those cases to closely parallel IV drug related AIDS cases.[3]

The Health and Human Services study previously cited also projected that by 1991 there would be at least ten to twenty thousand HIV infected children in the U.S., and it concluded that AIDS is now the number nine cause of death among children one to four years old.

Caregivers who treat chemically dependent women and their babies report a sad story. They note that AIDS progresses rapidly in babies, and they become very ill. Certain infections, when experienced by children, are much more severe than in adults. And children with AIDS also experience many neurological problems, brain diseases, seizures, motor dysfunction, and physical abnormalities.[4] Treatment programs in the Northeast report more than three-quarters of the AIDS cases in children under thirteen are acquired before birth, and more than one-half that number are born to IV drug users. In New York City, about 77 percent of children with AIDS are born to either IV drug users or sex partners of IV drug users.[5]

Given these numbers, it's essential that a woman considering pregnancy — whether she is already HIV positive or indulges in high-risk behaviors — be fully aware of the risks to her baby and to herself. She needs education about the risks of drug use and high-risk sexual behavior not only as it affects herself but how it might affect her baby. She needs to know how to stay healthy, how to change her lifestyle, how to take precautions to prevent transmission, and how to recognize the signs that are part of HIV related diseases.

She is also the best one to decide whether to continue the pregnancy, to terminate, or not to get pregnant in the first place. But she can make a far better decision for herself and her baby if she has complete and sympathetic counseling based on a clear knowledge of the risks under those conditions. Even with that knowledge, however, the decision to continue or discontinue a pregnancy due to fear of HIV infection can be agonizing for any parent.

Case History

Alice, an entertainer, fell deeply in love with her boss, a married man who regularly used IV drugs. When she became pregnant she feared her baby might be born with AIDS, but she very much wanted the child. John refused to be tested, but it was widely known that his wife had recently died of complications of AIDS.

Though Alice tested negative for HIV, she was afraid she still might be infected, as it occasionally takes time for antibody to the HIV virus to develop and show up on the test. But time was running out for a medically safe abortion to be done, if that was to be her choice.

So Alice's attorney, armed with a court order and threatening charges of attempted manslaughter, forced John to agree to a test. When it was revealed that John was indeed positive, Alice made the agonizing decision to continue the pregnancy. In her eighth month, Alice too converted to seropositive.

The antibody positive baby was born six weeks later, appearing healthy. But it will be a year and a half before it can be determined conclusively if the infant is really infected or is just showing anti-bodies that came from his mother.

Alice knows there is a fifty-fifty chance either way. She also knows that since she has no family members willing to care for them, if she becomes ill, there will be no one to care for the baby. Clearly the anxiety about her decision will be with Alice for some time.

Risk by Transfusion

For completeness sake, it should be mentioned that even with careful testing of all blood prior to tranfusion, a rare infected unit of blood may test negative. This blood may infect and cause AIDS in the recipient. There are no perfectly reliable tests of anything in the world. And while the blood supply today is safer than ever before, physicians doing elective surgery should encourage patients to minimize the use of tranfusions in favor of autologous blood — the patient's own blood banked in advance.

If Infected, What Are the Odds?

What if a patient or client becomes infected? What are their chances of getting AIDS? And if they get AIDS, what are their chances of survival?

It is very important to know, media reports aside, that most people who have been infected so far have not gotten AIDS, and many people with AIDS survive for a long time. AIDS is not 100 percent fatal.

Scientific studies show us that in certain groups of gay men studied, about 38 percent of those testing positive developed AIDS within six years.[6] That means 62 percent did not!

And while 90 to 95 percent of people diagnosed with AIDS in 1981 through 1982 have, according to the CDC, not survived, 5 to 10 percent remained alive six years later.[7] On the basis of a larger group of men studied in New York, it was projected that the probability of five year survival was 15 percent, and for gay men with Kaposi's sarcoma it was 30 percent.[8] That certainly is a long step away from the death sentence that AIDS was initially thought to be.

What may be promoting these improved survival rates is explored in more detail in Chapter Eleven.

ENDNOTES

1. D. R. Bolling and B. Voeller, "AIDS and Heterosexual Anal Intercourse," *Journal of the American Medical Association* vol. 258, no. 4 (24 July 1987): 474.

2. N. Padlan, et al., "Male to Female Transmission of Human Immunodeficiency Virus," *Journal of the American Medical Association* vol. 258, no. 6 (14 August 1987): 788.

3. R. M. Selik, et al., "Distribution of AIDS Cases by Racial/Ethnic Group and Exposure Category — United States, June 1, 1981 to July 4, 1988," *Morbidity and Mortality Weekly Report* vol. 37, Special Supplement no. 3 (1988): 1.

4. L. Finnegan, "Chemically Dependent Women, Their Children, And AIDS — A Workshop," in *Keeping Hope Alive*, Milan Korcok, ed. (Providence, Rhode Island: Manisses Communications, 1988): 47.

5. Ibid., 49.

6. J. E. Kaplan, et al., "A Six Year Followup of HIV Infected Homosexual Men With Lymphadenopathy," *Journal of the American Medical Association* vol. 260, no. 18 (11 November 1988): 2,694.

7. Larry Siegel, "AIDS: Perceptions versus Realities," *Journal of Psychoactive Drugs* vol. 20, no. 2 (April/June 1988): 149.

8. R. Rothenberg, et al., "Survival With the Acquired Immunodeficiency Syndrome," *New England Journal of Medicine* vol. 317, no. 21 (19 November 1987): 1,297.

CHAPTER FOUR

The Interface: AIDS and Drugs

To understand how alcohol and other drugs might pave the way for HIV infection or progression of HIV-related disease, it helps to probe the mysteries of our immune system and see how our defense mechanisms kick into action when threatened by invaders. Anyone with Pac Man experience will be able to visualize the scene quite clearly.

When a virus penetrates the skin and gets inside a person, it is first absorbed by a white blood cell that is like a sentry or guard, called a macrophage. The macrophage ordinarily either chews up invaders like HIV, or triggers a response from other, more sophisticated cells that have more weapons with which to kill the invader. That more sophisticated cell is the T-4 lymphocyte.

The T-4 lymphocyte in turn calls up another warrior cell, the "Natural Killer" lymphocyte to come join the battle. Under normal conditions, the T-4 cell and the N-K cell team up with the macrophage to knock out the invader.

That's what happens during the attack. But what if the cells that are directly assaulted by HIV are weakened even before the attack? What if they are made even more susceptible?

In AIDS, the signals and battle plans get crossed up, and HIV enters the battle with an invasion plan that knocks the T-4 cells, N-K cells and, to an extent, the macrophages themselves. This reversal opens up an opportunity for life-threatening infections to occur.

25

Alcohol, Other Drugs, and Immune Function

Studies have shown that even a few beers can make a person's T-4 cells twenty-five to two hundred fifty times more susceptible to HIV infection.[1] And it's been known for years that heavy alcohol use increases susceptibility to infectious disease, especially tuberculosis, klebsiella pneumonia, and other bacterial infections.

Because of the neurochemical similarities between alcohol and certain tranquilizers, particularly the benzodiazepines, HIV infected people should be cautious about using these drugs, though no research has been done to date to implicate them. Opiates, like heroin and its cogeners, also suppress the function of T-4 cells. Marijuana, while not studied well in humans, has been shown to directly suppress the ability of N-K cells to function in animals.[2, 3, 4, 5] And animal studies indicate that cocaine may be capable of speeding up the replication of HIV in already infected cells by up to 1,100 times.[6]

As for prescription medications, it has been reported that the susceptibility rate for HIV infection in women who use oral contraceptives is higher than in those who don't use them.

The direct effects of drugs on the immune system have been studied intermittently. And though no definite long-term effects on generalized immunity have been documented, acute effects have been noted. For example, it has been shown that atrophy of the thymus, which is the source of T-cells, occurs in rats fed alcohol; this same kind of atrophy also occurs in people with AIDS.

Analysis of T-cell subsets has also shown reduced T-4 cells in IV drug users compared to nonusers. And the correlation between use of nitrites (poppers) and development of Kaposi's sarcoma now seems more definable.[7]

Besides depletion of the T-4 cells, several other immunologic defects are commonly seen in persons with AIDS: reduced number and function of N-K cells, lowered amount or effect of interleukin 11 (important in activating the immune system to respond to invaders), and diminished function of T-8 cells. Many, if not all, of these anatomical changes and physiological reactions are also provoked by alcohol and other neuroactive drugs.

Disinhibition by Alcohol and Other Drugs

In addition to their direct effects on cellular structures, alcohol and other drugs influence behavior. Alcohol disinhibits its users. It sometimes allows and encourages them to drop their restraints and act out high-risk, dangerous behaviors they would never consider doing while sober.

Case History

Donald, age 31, entered his third rehabilitation program in as many years after relapsing back into his dependency on alcohol and other drugs. He had been diagnosed with AIDS and with Kaposi's sarcoma eight months earlier.

His open disclosure of AIDS to his counselor, his group, and the entire therapeutic community allowed a thorough exploration of his hatred of himself for being homosexual and of his "punishment" by contracting AIDS. The strong support he received in rehabilitation encouraged him to believe that he had the power and the option to "choose life" for himself, and he discovered a connection to a Higher Power, something very powerful, outside of himself, for the first time in his life.

After treatment he enthusiastically attended meetings of AA, Narcotics Anonymous (NA), and an HIV positive support group. He began to work part-time and he felt quite well.

Six months later, he still did not have a sponsor, nor was he actively working the Twelve Steps. But he assured his physicians and friends that he was doing fine.

Two months later, at a disco, he began drinking heavily and soon became involved in several sexual encounters with other men. He used no precautions and didn't tell them he had AIDS. Afterward, he was ashamed and contrite, but he had no recollection of the names of his sexual partners. He subsequently rejoined his AA group, but disclosed his guilt only to his physician.

Drugs and High-Risk Sex

Studies show a relationship between alcohol and other drug use and unsafe sex practices. In one study, 65 percent of gay men said they used alcohol or other drugs before or while they were having sex, and 18 percent said they got so drunk during these encounters they would not drive a car.[8]

Gay and bisexual men interviewed about their behaviors have said they are aware that they are more likely to have unsafe sex after they have used alcohol or drugs.[9] But it is unclear whether IV drug users, hemophiliacs, and other HIV positive individuals, who should consider themselves infectious to others, are similarly aware of such risks.

It's apparent that education about the risks of disinhibition might play a powerful role in containing the spread of AIDS, since alcohol and other drug use is widespread among people who engage in risky behaviors.

One study of clients in a large community-based organization of people with AIDS showed 100 percent of them used some alcohol or other drugs. In another study, compiled for the Centers for Disease Control, adult heterosexual AIDS patients who were not from so-called high-risk groups (they were not gay, not IV drug users, and not hemophiliacs) had all used marijuana. And of homosexual men in that study, 96 percent had used nitrites, 80 percent had used marijuana, 66 percent had used cocaine, and 50 percent had used ethyl chloride (that is similar in effect to "poppers"). Poppers are an inhalant form of nitrites used medically to dilate the blood vessels of the heart. They are used recreationally by drug users because they also dilate the blood vessels in the brain causing a rush of blood, described as "getting high."

Drug Use in the Gay Community

The prevalence of chemical abuse problems in the gay community is certainly a matter of great concern within the context of AIDS. A number of investigators have noted that drug use in the gay population is far more prevalent than it is in comparable heterosexual groups. There are many explanations for that.

Despite a greater openness about the subject of homosexuality over the past decade or two, a fear and loathing of people who are homosexual still exists throughout much of society. That unreasonable, irrational fear is called *homophobia*. And the fear exists even among many people who consider themselves enlightened.

Because of this fear, homosexuals are not as free to pursue personal, social, and sexual relationships as are heterosexuals. They are discriminated against. They don't have the same social outlets. Many respond to this lack by congregating in gay bars where they might be able to express themselves more freely.

Others resort to alcohol and other drugs in hope of making the world seem a less hostile, more accommodating place. And drugs open many pathways to behaviors that invite the transmission of HIV.

CD Caregivers Have Special Skills

Stopping the transmission of HIV urgently requires the intervention of chemical dependency treatment professionals, and for the application of compassionate, contemporary treatment methods.

The training and skills of caregivers experienced in dealing with stigma and denial are especially apt in treating persons with AIDS and dealing also with the special needs of HIV positive people. No other health care professionals come to this task so well prepared as those who specialize in chemical dependency treatment.

As many clinicians have already noted, treating chemical dependency in patients with HIV Spectrum Disease appears to have an overall salutary effect, benefiting not just the symptoms of dependency, but other symptoms as well. Treating chemical dependency eliminates exposure to immuno-suppressive drugs and improves nutrition. It encourages healthier lifestyles. It gets the individual into a drug-free environment that reduces the chances of repeated exposures to HIV, other viruses, bacteria, and parasites. It allows the opportunity for education about health and risk reduction. And it offers recourse to caregivers skilled in talking about life problems, family relationships, spirituality, and self-help — all issues that the person with HIV Spectrum Disease may have deep concerns about.

Certainly, Russ' story in Chapter Two emphasizes how a recovering HIV positive alcoholic can improve his or her chances of holding on to good health and fulfilling relationships if given the motivation to stay sober.

The Brain/Immune Connection

Clearly, the brain and the emotions have a compelling influence over the functioning of the body and its immune system. The study of these relationships, known as *psychoneuroimmunology*, is becoming increasingly important as a subject of research and clinical application — in terms of our knowledge of AIDS and drug use.

Direct connections between the brain and the immune system, specifically the T-cells, have been demonstrated. The mind and the body are connected — they talk to each other.[10] Many negative behaviors are associated with depression of the immune system; these behaviors occur in people who are chemically dependent, in people who are facing stressful situations, and in people who internalize fear. We are beginning to realize that enkephalins and other neurotransmitters that increase in the brain during recovery from chemical dependency may be enhanced by specific biobehavioral techniques, such as guided imagery, meditation, and mirror work (see page 34).

Whether direct intervention strategies of the kind used in chemical dependency recovery programs can positively alter the course of HIV Spectrum Disease remains to be seen, but the possibilities are enormous and very exciting.

ENDNOTES

1. O. Bagasra, et al., "Effects of Acute Alcohol Ingestion on In Vitro Susceptibility to Peripheral Blood Mononuclear Cells to Infection with Immunodeficiency Virus on Immune Function," *Proceedings of the Society for Experimental Biology and Medicine* (1987).

2. Larry Siegel, "AIDS: Relationship to Alcohol and Other Drugs," *Journal of Substance Abuse Treatment* 3 (1986): 271.

3. R. R. MacGregor, "Alcohol and Other Drugs as Co-factors for AIDS," *Advances in Alcohol and Substance Abuse* vol. 7, no. 2 (1987): 47.

4. H. Friedman, et. al., "Drugs of Abuse and Virus Susceptibility," in *Psychological, Neuro-psychiatric and Substance Abuse Aspects of AIDS,* T. P. Bridges, ed. (New York: Raven Press, 1988): 125.

5. R. R. Donohoe and A. Falek, "Neuroimmunomodulation by Opiates and Other Drugs of Abuse," in *Psychological, Neuropsychiatric and Substance Abuse Aspects of AIDS,* 145.

6. O. Bagasra and L. Formon, "Functional Analysis of Lymphocyte Subpopulations in Experimental Cocaine Abuse: 1. Dose Dependent Activation of Lymphocyte Subsets."

7. H. Haverkos and J. A. Dougherty, "Health Hazards of Nitrite Inhalants," *NIDA Research Monograph* (1988): 83.

8. R. R. MacGregor, "Alcohol and Other Drugs as Cofactors for AIDS," *Advances in Alcohol and Substance Abuse* vol. 7, no. 2 (1987): 47.

9. R. Stall, "The Prevention of HIV Infection Associated with Drug and Alcohol Use During Sexual Activity," *Advances in Alcohol and Substance Abuse* vol. 7, no. 2 (1987): 73.

10. G. F. Solomon, "Psychoneuroimmunology, AIDS and Chemical Dependency," in *Keeping Hope Alive*, Milan Korcok, ed. (Providence, Rhode Island: Manisses Communications, 1988): 15.

CHAPTER FIVE

Diagnosing and Counseling Persons with HIV Spectrum Disease

In the foreseeable future, all health care professionals will be asked to provide care for increasing numbers of people who are potentially HIV seropositive, have already been tested, want to be tested, or should be tested because of their high-risk behavior.

A Need to Counsel

The need to know about AIDS, and the need to counsel those who have it or are at high-risk for it, is particularly important for specialists in internal medicine, family practice, obstetrics/gynecology, psychiatry, and all caregivers in chemical dependency treatment. In fact, all professionals diagnosing or treating patients with a history of alcohol or other drug abuse, or high-risk sexual behaviors, should be prepared to provide appropriate counseling.

AIDS has been with us only a short time. While a few sporadic cases were recorded in the United States in the late 1970s, the epidemic dates back to 1981. The development of a vaccine or other medication that might prevent its spread is not imminent, although drugs such as zidovudine (formerly known as AZT or azidothymidine) have significantly improved the quality of life and survival times of those who can get these drugs and tolerate them.[1]

Educating All Staff and Patients

A complete pharmacological response to a complex, biopsychosocial disease such as AIDS is bound to take a long time. For now, the only proven way to prevent the spread of HIV infection and AIDS is by education. And no one is in a better position to provide that education than chemical dependency counselors and other health caregivers who deal every day with the complex biopsychosocial disease of addiction.

Basic information about the medical manifestations of AIDS should become part of the core knowledge of all physicians. And an awareness of the limited ways that HIV is spread, along with knowledge of the basic precautions necessary to prevent infection should be part of routine, daily educational processes of all chemical dependency counselors and treatment staff.

Everyone is afraid of AIDS, whether they are at risk or not. Admitting that fear and acknowledging that it is universal help put people on an equal footing when discussing AIDS. It's also a good first step in getting a productive dialogue going.

In addition to talking about the fear generated by AIDS, experiential exercises such as biofeedback, mirror work, and guided imagery are particularly useful in dealing with the negative emotions among treatment staff. Biofeedback is the process by which a reflex physiological response such as an increased heart rate due to fear, is controlled by conscious learned physical or mental exercises. Mirror work involves direct positive affirmations about oneself while in front of a mirror. Guided imagery is the development of strong, affirmative mental images created by a third person or by oneself on audiotape. These are powerful techniques to enhance immune function and a sense of well-being.

Recent studies indicate that many physicians and other caregivers are both judgmental and fearful about the people who have contracted AIDS or who are HIV positive, believing the patients are responsible for their own illness, that they have inflicted this condition upon themselves, and have only themselves to blame. These attitudes are not too different from that held by a good portion of society toward alcoholics and other drug addicts. It is, however, possible to overcome these attitudes.

Case History

Janet is a counselor in a hospital-based chemical dependency treatment program that has been openly accepting HIV positive patients, some with AIDS. The patients are fully integrated into the routine educational group therapy and therapeutic activities of the facility. HIV positive and HIV negative patients share the same rooms, the same washing machines, and go to AA meetings together.

Still, problems occasionally arise. Sometimes, an HIV negative patient insists not to sit next to an HIV positive person at the lunch table or in a van on the way to an AA meeting. This is dealt with in a matter-of-fact way by additional education and counseling of the recalcitrant patient. But separation is not allowed to continue.

The staff also gets regular updates on AIDS from the medical director and a specially trained nurse assigned part-time to the unit to monitor compliance with infectious disease precautions. The precautions are identical for all patients in the facility.

"In the beginning we were all terrified," says Janet of those first tentative steps toward integration of HIV positive patients. "We thought that being around an AIDS patient was dangerous, and certainly hugging, touching, or being around when they sneezed or coughed was inviting death on ourselves. No way could we see having them in our unit.

"Besides, we thought they would all die in a few months anyway so why bother trying to sober them up? Well, our medical director

attended a few seminars and then began to talk to us, all of us. Not just the counselors, but the nurses, the cleaning people, the food service people, everyone. And not just once, but every week or two for a while. Then, after he told us that being afraid was normal and okay, we decided we would face that fear directly.

"We got one of the cleaning people to act as a patient and one of the nurses to act as an AIDS nurse and we videotaped their interaction. The nurse was terriffic! You could tell she was afraid to go into the room and she avoided touching the patient the entire time. I mean, she put on gloves to check his blood pressure!

"The patient acted angry but resigned about the nurse's behavior. When we played the video, everyone could identify with one of the players. We talked about our feelings while watching the video and gradually we came to realize that it was our own fears of death and repugnance of discussing sexuality that were the real problem. We realized that we all had the feelings to one degree or another, including our AIDS patients.

"As we became increasingly aware of the realities of HIV transmission and talked openly about our fears, without anyone telling us that we should not be afraid, we became increasingly able to function normally even if the fear didn't go completely away. We learned how to protect ourselves from the blood of patients, and we knew that so long as no sex occurred and no blood was exchanged, we were safe.

"Today," Janet concludes, "we continue our regular sessions about AIDS, alcohol, and other drugs for patients and staff alike, on a regular basis. Lots of brochures and other educational materials are available. We support each other. We care. And we know we are making a difference."

When a person, whether a patient or caregiver, has fear of illness and does not respond rationally to education and counseling, it can be defined as a phobic reaction and may require specific therapeutic intervention. Such a reaction needs to be addressed; so does the fear of death and dying.

To deny patients and staff an opportunity to talk about their anxieties and fears of death, when many around them of their own ages are dying, is to avoid one of the major personal reactions to HIV infection.

Yet, everyone must admit that it's not easy to talk about such a painful subject. Many caregivers, especially physicians, are not used to sharing feelings. They suffer in silence. In the meantime, they see patients whom they may have helped through years of recovery from chemical dependency dying from AIDS. These are not burdens to be handled alone. Staff members need support to deal with them. And such support should be a part of routine in-service training.

Educating Families and Loved Ones

Family therapy has become a basic part of modern chemical dependency treatment. There are few programs now that fail to address the reality that chemical dependency is not an illness neatly contained in individual patients but is intertwined in the patient's family relationships.

Similarly, the family must be involved in the care of persons with HIV Spectrum Disease. This too is a condition that deeply affects family and friends. It too is laden with guilt, stigma, and hidden feelings.

The devastating circumstances are all too common as parents, wives, and children discover all at once that a loved one has AIDS and is chemically dependent.

Case History

Rob had been coughing — a dry, hacking, annoying cough that kept his lover, Tim, awake at night. The coughing went on for about a month before Rob finally went to the doctor. He also noticed he was having more and more trouble getting his breath when he rode his bike around town or went for a swim.

He was having to make lists to remember things like picking up the laundry or picking up batteries for the hurricane flashlights. He never needed lists before.

Tim was becoming increasingly upset that Rob wouldn't do anything to help himself and was still smoking pot every day or so, and smoking cigarettes as well. The smoking was driving Tim wild.

When Dr. Stone finished the exam and told Rob he would have to go to the hospital immediately for x-rays and a blood test, Rob knew. In spite of the bravado before Dr. Stone and Tim, he was terrified. He knew it was AIDS, though he had never been tested, and he knew he was going to die, and soon. No matter what they said!

Rob had lived with Tim for seven years but had never acknowledged being gay to his father, a fundamentalist minister, or to any other family member. He had cut off most family ties, only occasionally visiting for a day or so, always saying his design business prevented him from staying longer. And he always visited alone.

When the AIDS diagnosis was confirmed, "pneumocystis pneumonia," Rob's world began to crash around him. By now his condition had worsened and he was in the intensive care unit. Clearly his parents would have to be told he was very ill.

When Tim called the Reverend Beckwith and told him his son was very ill with a rare kind of pneumonia, he tried to be evasive. But finally he had to say that the doctor thought Rob might have AIDS. The silence on the other end of the line was deafening, but Mr. Beckwith finally said he would come.

On the layover in Atlanta, Mr. Beckwith spoke to one of his other sons who now also knew about the AIDS diagnosis. The son confided: "Dad, I think Rob is gay."

The shaken clergyman thought of all the years he preached about the "abomination" of homosexuality. A daughter with a child born out of wedlock, another drug-addicted son saved by prayer, and now this. "Maybe I should have been celibate," he said sorrowfully to Dr. Stone later.

He arrived at Rob's bedside, holding a large Bible and asking his now comatose son to renounce his homosexuality and be saved from damnation. He pointed a finger at the disconsolate Tim, standing with his mother at his side, and said, "You! You are my son's murderer."

Over the next days, Mrs. Beckwith and the other children came in one at a time. A truce was declared, unspoken but real. There was only a shared grief, a sense of deep loss of friendship, of losing a son and a brother, of years never to be retrieved.

When Rob died, the family left with their feelings not yet resolved. Tim sent Rob's remains back to Texas where they were buried quietly, without anyone saying exactly what had happened. Rob's belongings went to Tim, because he had willed them that way. But the bitterness remained. Five years passed. Tim found someone else, but he never spoke of Rob or his family. There has never been any contact since, either way.

Families, including extended families and significant others, need to be able to allay their apprehension about getting AIDS from a loved one. They need to have information presented clearly and persuasively. They need to know that no family member has ever developed AIDS or even become seropositive from touching, hugging, sharing eating utensils, or any other nonsexual, nonneedle sharing activity.

Intimate sexual partners of HIV positive persons must also know the risks they face and how to avoid them. They must be carefully counseled and educated about high-risk sexual activities, proper condom use, the need to stay healthy, and keeping their immune system strong and intact. More on risk reduction will be discussed in Chapter Eight.

Dealing with Grief

It's essential for the professional to understand the stages that all people go through as part of the grieving process — the shock and denial, anger or depression, bargaining, understanding, and finally accepting the inevitability and the loss.

It's equally important for AIDS and HIV positive patients and their families to understand the process of grieving, to recognize its stages, and to accept them as perfectly normal experiences that serve a very useful purpose in protecting them from further psychological damage.

Allowing the process to continue at an uninterrupted, but carefully monitored pace, with care to detect pathological behavior is the mark of a well-trained professional. The commonly held notion that denial is bad and requires immediate confrontation is a frequent counseling error.

Knowing When and Where to Refer

Not everyone who provides health care can deal with the AIDS or HIV infected patient, especially when the patient is also chemically dependent. That takes education and special skills. But all health caregivers should be able to recognize certain signs that show the possibility of HIV infection, and those that indicate chemical dependency. In confronting either, caregivers should be prepared to make an appropriate referral. If in doubt, ask a knowledgeable physician.

There are many subtle manifestations of HIV infection that should trigger our suspicions: seborrhea of the face and scalp; mild polyarthralgia or neuritis, including Bell's palsy or multidermatomal shingles; forgetfulness; persistent fungal infections of the skin; and other signs.

As for being aware to the possibility of chemical dependency — aside from its most obvious signs such as uncontrollable use of alcohol or other drugs — look for emotional instability, and a variety of compulsive behaviors such as overspending of money, intensive gambling, hypersexuality, overeating or anorexia, and legal infractions.

Certainly, by the time HIV has progressed to include weight loss, fever and diarrhea, or a dry nonproductive cough, the illness is already far along. Similarly, by the time the use of alcohol and other drugs has led to blackouts, absence from work, or physical abuse, the disease is well established.

If, for whatever reason, a health professional is unable to provide safe and effective care of the patient, there is an absolute ethical obligation to appropriately refer that patient.

Most larger communities now have AIDS related organizations that can assist with referrals. The U.S. Public Health Service AIDS hot line number is 1-800-342-AIDS.

ENDNOTES

1. T. Creagh-Kirk et al., "Survival Experience Among Patients with AIDS Receiving Zidovudine," *Journal of the American Medical Association* vol. 260, no. 20 (20 November 1988): 3,009.

CHAPTER SIX

Treating AIDS and Chemically Dependent Patients

As the AIDS epidemic spread and overlapped into large populations of drug users, their partners, and children, the need for all chemical dependency treatment caregivers to learn about AIDS and HIV transmission became critical.

HIV in Drug Users and Partners

As early as 1982, epidemiological projections made at the Haight-Ashbury Free Medical Clinics in San Francisco showed AIDS would soon exact a heavy toll among IV drug users. Subsequent studies in other areas such as New York, verified what those early projections only hinted at.

Now it has become clear that a majority of IV drug users being admitted to many chemical dependency treatment programs, especially in the Northeast, are HIV positive.

Chemical dependency programs should regard all patients as potentially HIV positive until proven otherwise. First, variable rates of seroconversion time exist (some become HIV positive shortly after exposure, others may take many months). Second, many are reluctant to consent to an HIV test. This makes it important not only for treatment staff to learn about AIDS, but to integrate that knowledge into their work. That means talking about and dealing with such emotionally charged issues as homophobia, mortality (one's own as well as the patient's), and sexual activity. Comfort with these issues isn't easily learned or easily addressed. All are highly intertwined with one's own subjective feelings.

Before beginning to treat patients, all caregivers should examine their own skills and attitudes carefully. They must be careful to balance the need for caution with the goal of aiding the patient's recovery.

Dealing with Your Feelings

One of the major barriers to effective management of AIDS patients is the attitude that they will all soon die and that everyone with a positive HIV test is going to "get it." If that is assumed, then the impediments to treatment are enormous. And if the caregiver has a deeply held, perhaps unconscious repugnance of homosexuality, IV drug users, or the contagion of death, there's the risk these feelings may be transferred to the patient, with an unfortunate result.

These personal, highly subjective attitudes may surface in benign ways. For example, the treatment professional may behave in an overly supportive, overly sympathetic, perhaps even patronizing way that is different from the clear, direct, more confrontational approach taken with other patients. Such a deviation will be noticed by the patient.

A good question to ask yourself is: *Am I treating this patient the same way I would treat an alcoholic woman who recently underwent a mastectomy for breast cancer?*

It is important for professionals to check out their own psychological state with colleagues. An especially effective way to do this is through discussions with a peer group, or perhaps as part of an in-service program. Increasingly, such activities are becoming part of the continuing training and education processes of chemical dependency programs.

Many physicians believe that persons with AIDS are personally culpable for their disease. To a large extent so are many cardiac or cancer patients, but since AIDS carries a stigma that the other diseases don't, the sense of culpability is aggravated.

Fear of Contagion

Nurses, chemical dependency counselors, and other caregivers are sometimes afraid that the AIDS patient poses grave and unusual threats to their safety and well-being. They fear that a hug in a group session carries contagion. The story told by Janet in Chapter Five shows just how deeply that fear might run through a professional staff faced for the first time with AIDS and HIV positive patients.

None of these fears is justified, especially if treatment programs put into place the Universal Blood and Body Fluid Precautions drawn up by the Centers for Disease Control and described fully in Chapter Seven. These precautions are now required by many accrediting and licensing agencies that inspect and regulate the quality standards of treatment units. With these in place, the risks of infection by normal therapeutic contact are virtually eliminated.

Preventing Infection in Treatment

The Universal Precautions are not extraordinary. They're not bizarre. They are the same precautions followed to prevent infection of other diseases such as hepatitis B. They can be easily applied. What's necessary are not more stringent precautions, space age uniforms, or aerosols to disinfect the air; what's needed is continuing education, done repeatedly, persuasively, and enthusiastically for all staff members. This education needs to be extended as often as necessary to keep abreast of new, emerging information.

Such education should exclude no one in the treatment environment. It should include clinical, administrative, and housekeeping personnel in hospitals, freestanding treatment centers, and office settings. It should be done to engage the interest and the mind, in language and with messages the intended audiences can understand, absorb, and identify with. Unabsorbed messages are useless. Spraying educational messages from on high by pompous lecturers using twenty-five cent rather than nickel words is, indeed, poor communication.

It is the professional's responsibility to ensure that the information has been heard, assimilated, and understood. Videotapes made in-house with your staff can be inexpensive yet effective educational tools. But they need to be available and readily used, by night staff as well as by the day shift. And they need to be used repeatedly to reinforce their messages, to maintain interest.

There is also a great need for education to clarify and correct the messages being put out daily, almost hourly, in the general media. No doubt that the general media has been instrumental in sensitizing the world to the gravity of AIDS. It has also precipitated much of the social, political, and even medical responses to the epidemic. But the media has also spread many myths and misleading generalizations. These need to be countered and exposed, and in-house education programs need to offer that opportunity.

Only when the staff is fully prepared is the facility ready to care for the patient with AIDS. If that preparation is not in place, if staff try to deal with AIDS on an ad hoc, impromptu, emotional basis, there is the potential for great damage.

Staff must be aware too that AIDS is an illness of fluctuating intensity and severity. Most HIV positive persons are totally asymptomatic. They look like anyone else, with no distinguishing clinical signs or features. And when symptoms do begin to occur, they might range from mild, flu-like aches and pains and low-grade fever, to quite severe illnesses such as life-threatening pneumonia, wasting diarrhea, opportunistic infections, or tumors.

The illness may also fluctuate in intensity in the same

individual over time, with periods of remission and relative good health reoccurring.

Differentiating AIDS from CD Symptoms

Differentiating neurocognitive impairment caused by AIDS from that caused by drugs is a common need in chemical dependency treatment settings. While the concept of dual diagnosis is familiar to chemical dependency professionals, the unique characteristics of neurocognitive impairment due to AIDS are not. And there are important distinctions to make.

Central nervous system disease in AIDS is often extremely subtle and may show up only as some mild, short-term memory loss. People may complain about forgetting phone numbers or grocery lists. They may have to write everything down — something they have not had to do before.

The amnesic spells (blackouts) of acute alcoholism or sedative use are not characteristic of AIDS. When they show up, they should indicate a chemical dependency problem.

The memory deficit associated with AIDS will frequently progress regardless of treatment. Memory deficit attributable to alcoholism or other drug abuse, on the other hand, will improve with abstinence from drugs. Other forms of impairment such as mild expressive aphasia (failure to understand language), or global loss of affect (a generalized lack of response to one's environment), are sometimes seen in AIDS patients, but when they occur in a chemically dependent person, they usually subside after the person is detoxified.

Acute anxiety and depression are very common in both AIDS and alcoholism and other drug dependency, but both are amenable to appropriate counseling.

Acute psychiatric manifestations of cerebritis (inflammation of the brain resulting in altered mental or neurological functioning), including psychotic states are sometimes seen in AIDS patients and may be extremely difficult to differentiate from the encephalopathy, or brain disease, caused by many drugs. Since a majority of current AIDS patients have histories of past or current alcohol or psychoactive drug abuse, that differentiation is best made after the effects of psychoactive drugs have worn off.

In this respect, the common practice of not making a psychiatric diagnosis of coincident bipolar (manic depressive) or affective disorder until well into the recovery phase of treatment may be well justified.

One must be careful, however, not to overlook opportunistic infections of the brain, most commonly those due to cryptococcus or toxoplasmosis, or central nervous system tumors such as primary lymphoma. In doing such investigations, CT or Magnetic Resonance Imaging scans, followed by lumbar puncture, are most useful and can be done with relatively little risk. Scans are also helpful in delineating so called "AIDS dementia" where cortical atrophy may be seen.

Clearly, treating the AIDS or HIV positive patient in the chemical dependency setting requires an increasingly broad range of skills and sensitivities. It also demands aggressive, educational efforts whose messages are clear, concise, presented in culturally relevant language, and are repeated over and over. Perhaps the most important of these messages is that with AIDS, as with chemical dependency, recovery is possible.

Professional caregivers should always offer hope.

CHAPTER SEVEN

Infection Control Precautions

Because it is almost impossible to predict with certainty who is or is not infected with HIV, the safest possible course in treating chemically dependent patients — or any other patients, — is to assume that all are HIV seropositive.

Assuming All Patients Are Positive

Certainly there are identifiable high-risk groups that come easily to mind. In San Francisco, between 50 and 75 percent of homosexual men tested are HIV positive. Of IV drug users in New York, 60 to 80 percent have tested positive.[1]

But it is also true that approximately 4 percent of unscreened trauma patients at some hospitals turn out to have been HIV positive,[2] and a smaller but significant percentage of military recruits are also showing evidence of prior exposure when tested.

The Virus Can Hide and Change

One of the more disturbing discoveries revealed recently is that minute amounts of HIV are being detected, by new techniques such as polymerase chain reaction (PCR), in blood test samples that don't show measurable antibody levels. One explanation for this may be that HIV can hide from antibody forming B-cells inside macrophages or possibly in stem cells. Or perhaps it's the very rapid mutation of the virus that keeps it from being readily detected.

What this means is that undetected infection may be lurking for a long time in places we don't suspect. This makes it necessary to assume that all patients are potentially infectious to others. The wisest course, therefore, is to use the CDC's Universal Precautions (described in Appendix One) when handling blood or other potentially infectious body fluids. Use of Universal Precautions in health care settings is the same kind of precaution that condoms and clean needles are for everyone.

The Centers for Disease Control, and infectious disease experts from around the world, agree that the Universal Precautions do not apply to feces, nasal secretions, sputum, sweat, tears, urine, or vomit unless they contain visible blood. The risk of transmission of HIV from these materials is extremely low or nonexistent.

Little Risk of Infection in Households

Studies have tried to determine the risk of infection in domestic situations where people with AIDS live. They have found that routine daily contact does not increase infection; it takes blood or sexual secretions containing HIV in adequate amounts to enter a person's body for infection to occur.

When this type of information, well substantiated and presented, is repeated as part of a treatment center's continuing staff education, as was reported earlier in Chapter Five, it can have a clearly stabilizing effect on treatment.

Little Risk to Health Care Workers

Thousands of health care workers, including doctors, nurses and lab technicians, have had direct exposure to infected blood-containing fluids in emergency rooms, surgical, or intensive care units, or laboratories since concern about AIDS emerged in the early 1980s. As of mid-1988, according to CDC surveillance of these cases, only seventeen individ-- uals have seroconverted on the basis of this exposure.[3]

Hugging, shaking hands, drinking out of the same glass, using the same clothes washer, using the same bathroom, swimming in a pool, or soaking in a hot tub does not transmit HIV. People with HIV can participate in group therapy, go to meetings of Twelve Step groups, participate in athletic activi- ties, meditation, exercises, and other activities with absolute safety to themselves and others.

Still, despite the low probability of HIV transmission in a domestic setting, it is a good idea for the HIV positive person to avoid exposure to potentially harmful organisms such as toxoplasmosis in cats and psittacosis in birds. So avoid clean- ing up the excrement, which may harbor these organisms. It's best to let a trained professional take care of diseased pets.

And because activation of the T-lymphocyte may cause increased activity or replication of HIV, HIV positive people should be careful to avoid exposure to additional viral or antigenic microorganisms such as intestinal parasites in moldy foods kept in refrigerators.

Finally, we should emphasize again that susceptibility to HIV infection, or its progression in people already infected, is at least partially controllable by them. There are many things people can do to influence their own immune status. The effects of alcohol and other drugs, specifically marijuana, opiate narcotics (whether from the street or the pharmacy), and cocaine can compromise parts of the immune system. This point must be made clear: those who use these drugs risk depressing their immune systems and making themselves vulnerable to successful attack by a number of diseases, in- cluding AIDS.

Nutrition, Moderation, and Immunity

One positive and easy step to immunocompetence is good nutrition. A good diet including adequate quantities of vitamins and minerals is essential. Yet counseling patients about nutrition is often overlooked. Caregivers, including primary care physicians, are often not comfortable talking about nutrition. It takes time. It takes repeating. Most medical and nursing schools don't give much time or emphasis to teaching nutrition. Yet it's very important for the HIV positive person to maintain proper nutritional support.[4] A good resource to recommend to patients is *Living with AIDS: Reaching Out*, by Tom O'Connor with Ahmed Gonzalez-Nunez.

One hypothesis for the increased prevalence of HIV Spectrum Disease and AIDS in Africa, Haiti, and the sugar cane and farming area around Belle Glade, Florida, is that the poor level of nutrition, substandard living quarters, and other environmental factors — any of which might damage the immune system — promote infection and the spread of disease.

The best advice for people who test positive for HIV, or who are chemically dependent, or who have AIDS, or who come into contact with a patient's body fluids, is not different from that which should guide everyone: eat well, don't drink, don't drug. Caregivers can further offer the advice so many recovering people have already learned in the AA slogan, HALT. Don't get Hungry, Angry, Lonely, or Tired.

ENDNOTES

1. C. R. Schuster, "NIAAA/NADA Research on Alcohol and Drug Abuse and AIDS — Current Projects and Future Needs," in *Keeping Hope Alive*, Milan Korcok, ed. (Providence, Rhode Island: Manisses Communications): 47.

2. G. D. Kelen et al., "Unrecognized Human Immuno-deficiency Virus Infection in Emergency Department Patients," *New England Journal of Medicine* vol. 318, no. 25 (23 June 1988): 1,645.

3. R. Marcus et al., "Surveillance of Health Care Workers Exposed to Blood from Patients Infected with the Human

Immunodeficiency Virus," *New England Journal of Medicine* vol. 319, no. 17 (27 October 1988): 1,118.

4. Tom O' Connor with Ahmed Gonzalez-Nunez, *Living with AIDS: Reaching Out* (San Francisco: Corwin Publishers, 1986).

CHAPTER EIGHT

Avoiding High-Risk Behavior

It can't be emphasized too often: infection by HIV does not occur casually or easily. And though there are certain factors such as drug use or accompanying disease that may predispose an individual to infection, there are also clear ways to prevent it.

If certain behaviors are avoided, the risks of exposure and infection do not occur. And since there is no "magic bullet," pill, or vaccine available today to prevent or cure AIDS, the key to avoiding it depends on altering high-risk behaviors.

The caregiver providing chemical dependency or other health services to HIV seropositive people, or those who might become infected, has a responsibility to try to change behaviors that put patients at risk. And that is so whether their patients are presenting symptoms of cardiovascular disease, diabetes, alcoholism, or AIDS.

What are these behaviors? How does a caregiver recognize them? What is the treatment for them?

Determining High-Risk Behaviors

For a body fluid to be infectious to others it must contain cells that contain virus. These blood cells — lymphocytes and/or macrophages (which are monocytes located in tissues) — must contain HIV and get into the body of another person in order to cause infection. This is the reason that blood, semen, and, to a lesser degree, cervical secretions in women, are the fluids implicated in viral transmission; because these fluids contain cells that contain virus. Thus, any behaviors that allow for passage of any body fluid containing white blood cells are at high risk for causing infection.

Because the rectal mucosa is far more fragile and less well lubricated than the vagina, unprotected rectal intercourse (without a condom and nonoxynol 9) is the most common mode of transmission of AIDS in the United States. And because this behavior is most common among gay men, this group has been hardest hit by the AIDS epidemic. Studies show that up to 25 percent of heterosexual women practice rectal intercourse occasionally, and up to 10 percent do so regularly.[1] This has implications for the spread of HIV.

Because rectal intercourse often involves tearing of tissue and, consequently, bleeding, it is a high-risk behavior. When large numbers of women practice such a behavior at the same time as the pool of HIV seropositive among both men and women continues to grow, the numbers at risk are greatly multiplied. It's thus apparent that there are more heterosexual women potentially at risk for HIV transmission via anal sexual intercourse than there are homosexual men.

Counseling Clearly and Effectively

In counseling patients, it's essential to understand the fundamental purpose of communications: the patient or client must *understand* what is being communicated. When professionals try to communicate with lay people, they too often fail because they don't put themselves in the place of those hearing what they are saying.

It's essential to talk simply, clearly, to repeat the message, and to do so in language the patient understands. That doesn't mean patronizing the patient with phoney and affected lingo. It means using whatever language, pictures, gestures, or ideas to get the message across.

In fighting the AIDS epidemic, we have placed most of our

trust in the value of preventive education. It's the best defense we have to date. But in many respects we have failed. Analyses of various AIDS brochures designed for high-risk groups show that the language used is at the second year college level.[2] And some are written at the first year graduate school reading level. This is not going to help most AIDS patients in America's inner cities — some of whom have had little or no education. It's not going to help those who have had even a moderate amount of education.

If gay men refer to anal intercourse as "ass fucking" or "getting fucked," that's the language to use when counseling them. Hispanics may use another term; blacks another.

It's not easy for professionals in a health care setting to talk about "fucking" to their patients. It takes practice, and sometimes it may help for the care giver to go to lectures by sex therapists or do some role playing with colleagues.

A good technique to build up confidence and comfort for such counseling is to sit together with peers, putting all the "dirty words" on a blackboard, saying them out loud, testing questioning techniques on each other, and allowing the counselors' problems with the language to be confronted and defused. In fact, this is little different from learning how to deal with other unpleasant issues, such as death and dying, or cancer in children.

It's also important not to assume too much about patients' knowledge of their own bodies and how they work. Some simple anatomy drawings and illustrations may be useful in counseling and teaching sessions.

Discussing Safer Sex

Advocating condom use is one thing. But discussing and describing how to use a condom properly and safely is quite another. The spermicidal material, nonoxynol 9, available over the counter in tubes, or sometimes already applied to condoms, can be used as a lubricant and it also kills HIV easily. (Specific instructions on condom use are in Appendix Two).

When condoms and other protective materials such as spermicides are used, previously unsafe sex practices become safer, but not totally safe because there is always the risk of a failure; it's estimated there is a 10 percent failure rate for these protective mechanisms. Thus, you should avoid the term "safe" sex. It may be safer with the appropriate precaution, but safety can never be considered an absolute. There are degrees of safety; nothing is 100 percent safe.

Unprotected vaginal intercourse also allows for cells containing virus to pass between men and women, both ways. But it's now thought that transmission from men to women is done more easily than transmission from women to men.

Taking a History

Just as important as the use of clear, explicit language in counseling, is the need for taking a careful history by talking about specific sexual practices. This must be done in a nonconfrontational, nonjudgmental way if any valid, reliable information is to be gained.

A question put calmly and directly is an inoffensive and effective way to get to the truth. For example, "Do you have sexual intercourse with women?" "Do you use a rubber condom?" "Do you put your penis into your partner's vagina, rectum?" Or even, "Do you use the front hole or the back hole?" If you ask these questions without using body language or intimidating vocal mannerisms that betray discomfort and negative attitudes, you can get a lot of reliable information.

Risks of Needle Sharing

Another way that HIV can enter the body is by direct injection of virus. Because there is a very high prevalence of

HIV in the blood of intravenous drug users, the sharing of injection equipment, needles, and syringes that have not been properly cleaned is extremely hazardous. The use of sterile, cleansed equipment for injection substantially reduces this risk of infection, but it certainly does not eliminate risk.

Intravenous drug use is not restricted to one group or "class" of people; it has been widely reported that the problem also exists among medical professionals.

The common use of sterile disposable equipment by IV drug-using physicians and nurses essentially protects them from infection by HIV, hepatitis B, and other infections transmissible by sharing blood-contaminated equipment. But few have such easy access to clean works as have health professionals.

Particularly on the West Coast, sharing equipment has a sexual connotation that helps addicts get high. But knowledge of HIV transmission has cut back on this practice.[3]

Needle sharing in the New York City area is also quite common, but has been attributed mostly to the economic fact that sharing is cheaper rather than that sharing is akin to a sexual experience.

Another notion, that IV drug users are not concerned about their own or their partner's drug use or sexual health also appears misguided. They do care. Otherwise, the marked reduction of needle sharing and the increase in proper needle cleaning that has been seen in San Francisco, for example, would not have occurred.

Where well-targeted, educational programs, using culturally relevant materials prepared in understandable language, are presented by trusted individuals — especially peers — behaviors can be changed.[4]

Educational Outreach

Outreach programs in New York, New Jersey, San Francisco, and other places have been credited with increasing proper condom use, decreasing needle sharing, and increasing the use of bleach and other disinfectants to keep needle equipment clean.

Outreach efforts, mostly by recovering addicts and peers of drug users, have also been instrumental in high density AIDS areas, like New Jersey and New York, in bringing drug using HIV infected persons into chemical dependency treatment.[5] Such efforts must be intensified. To give up on trying to modify behaviors, and to give in to mandatory testing and quarantining of all HIV seropositive people, is to throw in the towel.

Certainly, if all people at risk said no to drugs and sex, the spread of HIV would virtually stop. But widespread compliance with such admonitions is not likely. As we have seen with cigarette smoking, cholesterol reduction, and other health risk reduction programs, modification of deep-seated behaviors is incremental, and there is often a good deal of relapse that accompanies it.

Risk behavior reduction for HIV, like relapse prevention for drugs and alcohol in treatment programs, is a process, not a "single moment of clarity." In counseling persons at risk, it's essential to point out that there are many drugs capable of suppressing the immune system and capable of acting as cofactors in the transmission of HIV and the spread of AIDS. And it isn't always extreme or bizarre use of these drugs that precipitates a high-risk situation.

For example, if a teenager gets high on a given drug, drops his or her defenses against careless sex, and happens to be with someone who is HIV positive and similarly disinhibited, the risks of infection increase enormously. Sex with somebody who is HIV positive becomes even more dangerous if drug use — even what is considered social use — suppresses the immune system, thus increasing susceptibility to any and all infections.

Since we are never certain who has the virus, the need for precautions is universal and comprehensive.

One unyielding precaution when having sex is to use condoms with nonoxynol 9 and to use them every time, from start to finish. There is nothing discretionary about that decision; it should be automatic.

Similarly, following universal precautions when providing health care to people, are absolutely essential. Every time. No exceptions.

ENDNOTES

1. D. R. Bolling, B. Voeller, "AIDS and Heterosexual Anal Intercourse," *Journal of the American Medical Association* vol. 258, no. 4 (24 July 1987): 474.

2. M. Hochhauser, "Health Planning for Chemically Dependent AIDS/ARC Patients," in *Keeping Hope Alive,* ed, Milan Korcok (Providence, Rhode Island: Manisses Communications, 1988), 78.

3. D. Smith, "Integrating AIDS Education and Treatment With Chemical Dependency Treatment," in *Keeping Hope Alive* , 69.

4. Ibid.

5. Joyce Jackson, "Integrating AIDS Education and Treatment With Chemical Dependency Treatment," in *Keeping Hope Alive* , 62.

CHAPTER NINE

HIV Antibody/Antigen Testing

HIV testing is a highly emotional issue that forces tough choices on patients and health care providers alike. Since AIDS was first discovered, the effort to find reliable and practical means to test for the presence of HIV has been vigorous. There are many who see testing for HIV as the most reliable way of screening and identifying persons who have been exposed to the AIDS virus and may be at risk for developing AIDS or infecting others. Some feel it is primarily by testing that we will be able to control the spread of the epidemic. Already, there have been several attempts by state and federal legislators to force mandatory tests on various populations such as hospital patients, pregnant women, couples applying for marriage licenses, prison inmates, and others. Bills have been drafted, but not passed, that would isolate all who tested positive and consign them to quarantine.

It's unrealistic to expect that such massive mandatory measures would control the spread of the AIDS epidemic, even if they were not so horrendously expensive, probably wasteful, and certainly insensitive to the rights of most citizens.

What HIV Tests Show and Don't Show

The Enzyme-Linked Immunosorbent Assay (ELISA), which tests for the presence of antibodies to HIV in serum or plasma, came into widespread use as a means of screening the nation's supply of blood and blood products. Since then it has been used widely in clinical settings to determine who has been exposed to HIV. But the ELISA only detects antibody to the HIV; it does not detect the live infectious virus — the organism that invades the body and generates the production of antibodies. It tells us only if the AIDS virus has been present. It does not diagnose AIDS. It is, in effect, a "footprint" that reveals the HIV virus has been present. It cannot confirm that the individual being tested can infect others or will go on to develop AIDS or other HIV spectrum diseases.

As a screening measure, ELISA results can't always be taken at face value in testing people who fear they may have been exposed to HIV, or in doing epidemiological studies of specific population groups. False positive results are not uncommon.

Some studies have shown that over 90 percent of positive results in low-risk populations are false.[1] Generally, at least two or three tests on the same serum should be done, and then positive results should further be confirmed with a virus-specific test such as the Western Blot. This test detects antibodies to multiple viral antigens.

The Indirect Immunofluorescence Assay (IFA) is another effective confirmatory test when done by experienced people, but it is not used as widely as the Western Blot.

The development of antibody and antigen tests to detect and confirm HIV is a burgeoning industry. But most of the tests under development are still available largely only in large medical centers, and they remain too expensive for broad screening purposes. Even the widely used ELISA test, when used to repeat an apparent positive result and followed up by a confirmatory Western Blot, costs between fifty and one hundred dollars. The other laboratory tests cost several times that apart from costs for pre- and post-test counseling.

When the ELISA antibody test was developed, it was seen as a major breakthrough that would help contain the spread of the epidemic — another procedure physicians could call on to make a diagnosis of AIDS, just as they rely on a urine test for blood sugar when screening for diabetes. But this was not to be. Not only does the HIV antibody test have technical limitations, but its use without proper knowledge of the possible implications, without clear consent of the person being tested, and without the strictest regard for confidentiality of results, has the potential for doing great damage to the person being tested.

The Need for Test Confidentiality

In chemical dependency programs, the need to keep a patient's admission and treatment record confidential is of the highest priority. Irreparable damage might be done to a person's reputation, career, and social life if revelations about his or her alcoholism or other drug addiction fall into unqualified or unauthorized hands. But with so many parties involved in the provision of health care services and benefits — insurance companies, employers, HMOs, utilization reviewers, and other "gatekeepers" — keeping data confidential is a tough job. There are a lot of people claiming a right to know all of the details about their employees or insurance beneficiaries.

There has been a great decrease in stigma about seeking treatment for alcoholism or other drug dependency. But a lot of stigma remains. And there are still many employers and insurers who do not accept addiction as an illness and would rather fire or drop persons with drug problems than provide them with health benefits.

Just as chemically dependent people have suffered from such discrimination, AIDS patients and HIV positive persons are even more damaged by discrimination.

Case History

To Patricia, settling down as an eighth grade teacher in a small community and remaining drug free for three years was a source of satisfaction and pride. Life was all she envisioned it could be when she decided to leave New York City and her IV drug world behind.

Part of the new life was a new boyfriend, thoughts of marriage, and having a baby. Diversions such as the cramping pain in her side, attributed by her doctor to gallstones, didn't intrude on her plans. During the summer holidays, the gallstones would be removed.

While in the operating room, however, a nurse who was passing instruments looked casually at Patricia's chart. She discovered the positive results of HIV tests ordered by the surgeon, done routinely by him without any special consent from, or knowledge by, his patients.

After an uneventful few days of recovery, Patricia returned home to find a letter from her school principal telling her she could not return to work because she had AIDS. When the story was fully told, the nurse admitted that she had called the school board with the HIV information because her own child was in the same school. She did not want her child to get AIDS from the teacher.

Patricia was suddenly unemployable. Her boyfriend no longer called. The health insurance ran out. A lengthy, highly publicized legal proceeding finally won her back pay and reinstatement to her job, but life would never be the same.

She began to drink heavily. One afternoon she got drunk, crashed through a plate glass window at the bar, and severed every artery in her right wrist.

Only her parents attended the funeral.

The decision of a patient to test for HIV status is a difficult and complex one, involving potential benefits to the patient's own treatment plan as well as to the public health. But it also involves enormous risks if the information is used wrongly or is inadequately interpreted or understood.

Most professional health care groups who have considered the pros and cons of testing agree on certain basic ground rules:

- Testing for HIV antibody should never be done without adequate counseling and clearly defined consent.

- Testing should only be done where the risks and benefits of the test to the person being tested or to those who might be infected by that person are clearly understood.
- Confidentiality of results must be protected.

A test should be done only after patients have been thoroughly counseled about what the test does and does not mean, how a positive test might affect them and their friends and family, how it might affect them and others psychologically, and how it might demand changes in the way they live.

Suppose a person's positive HIV test result has leaked from a hospital, chemical dependency unit, or public health agency into an insurer's hands. It's very unlikely that he or she will get health, life, or disability insurance.

If the information comes to the attention of a potential employer, will that person get the job? And how might it affect the existing employer and the people with whom this person has worked for years?

And how will that information influence the person's landlord, dentist, eye doctor, teachers, and everyday social contacts? Look how it affected Patricia!

The Need to Protect Against Discrimination

The New York State Department of Health recently drafted a recommended consent form for HIV Antibody Testing in which clear and simple language states what the the person considering taking a test should think about before giving written approval for it. After outlining what the HIV antibody shows or does not show, the consent form says that knowledge of test results might help doctors treat patients for certain illnesses such as tuberculosis. It may also help patients make some personal decisions about the way they live and the risks they represent for others.

The consent form also notes that if a person tests positive and others learn of that result, they may be discriminated against by neighbors, friends, family, employers, landlords, insurance companies, and others. Therefore, says the consent form, people should be "extremely careful in disclosing their test results to anyone."

The form states that help is available through the State Division of Human Rights and the New York City Commission on Human Rights to investigate and prosecute those who illegally discriminate against HIV infected persons. These safeguards are often not available in other states, however.

Infection Control in Treatment Centers

Because there has been so much focus on the relationship between drug use and HIV transmission, it's only normal to expect patients entering treatment for alcoholism or other drug abuse to be especially sensitive about their risks of contracting the HIV virus while in treatment.

They know that IV drug users are at particularly high-risk for HIV transmission. In some programs on the East Coast, more than 60 percent of IV drug users who have been tested have tested positive.[2]

The ratio of HIV positive people is so high in some of these areas that chemical dependency programs simply assume every IV drug user is positive, whether tested or not, and they apply appropriate infection control procedures to everyone, as should be the case in all health care settings.

Since these procedures are no different from those required to prevent the spread of other transmissible disease, such as hepatitis B, and since they are already recommended as routine procedures for all health care facilities, their application simplifies and enhances infection disease control. Universal precautions are now required by the Joint Commission on Accreditation of Health Care Organizations (JCAHO) and the Occupational Safety and Health Administration (OSHA).

Nonetheless, people entering chemical dependency treatment are, except maybe for their specific addiction, no different from other patients — they have fear and anxiety; chances are they have not been well-informed about AIDS; and their instincts often overcome their intellect.

Many workers, students, and even patients in chemical dependency or other treatment centers are not comfortable with the thought they may be living or working next to drug users or alcoholics who may have a period of IV drug use hidden in their background. Perhaps they have also heard that people whose immune systems are suppressed by alcohol or other drugs are at higher than normal risk for carrying the virus.

They may feel safe knowing everyone about them has been tested and only those proven negative have been allowed through the doors. As noted previously, however, because of the problem of false positive and false negative results, this sense of safety may be misguided.

Because of the high relationship between drug use and HIV positivity and AIDS, some groups and legislators want all patients entering chemical dependency programs to be tested for HIV. And certainly, such testing would allow compilation of a lot of interesting epidemiology about HIV prevalence among drug users. But there is also great danger in opening the floodgates to the many other problems we've already discussed. Health care professionals should always consider the individual patient's circumstances and needs before doing any procedure, including HIV testing.

Benefits of HIV Testing

Knowledge of a patient's HIV status is particularly useful in preventing and treating tuberculosis, syphilis, and certain varieties of pneumonia — infections which thrive in the presence of suppressed immune response.

Since HIV Spectrum Disease is essentially caused by the

body's failure to maintain an adequate immune defense, such infections need to be monitored with special care and may need to be treated more aggressively than they would in a person with normal immune function. Knowledge of HIV positive status helps maintain that vigilance.

Already there is plenty of evidence that prevalence of such infections is on the increase in populations with a high incidence of drug addiction and HIV seropositivity. Studies done in New York City, where the crossover between HIV positivity and intravenous drug use is especially high, show that since the onset of the AIDS epidemic, deaths from other infectious diseases such as endocarditis, tuberculosis, and bacterial pneumonias have increased sharply.[3]

Knowing one's HIV status can also help guide certain intervention or prevention activities. For example, a woman who learns she is positive for HIV antibody might want to consider abortion early in pregnancy.

An HIV positive patient who would otherwise be a candidate for some form of immunosuppressive therapy — as in an organ transplantation or artificial insemination — could be given other options.

We can also hope that people who know they are HIV positive would do everything in their power to protect themselves from compounding their risk by eliminating dangerous behaviors such as drug use and unsafe sex, and by enhancing their health through sound nutrition, moderate living, exercise, and adequate rest.

And with the development of medications such as zidovudine (previously called AZT, known by its trade name Retrovir™) and other experimental therapies showing themselves capable of preventing the progression of HIV related illness, it is increasingly useful to know one's HIV status. If intervention with these new medications can halt or slow the disease process from HIV infection to AIDS, there will be a tremendous motivation among people in the high-risk behavior groups to find out their HIV status and deal with it.

Risks of Testing

The major risk of being tested for HIV is that the results may fall into the wrong hands. There is no scarcity of horror stories about HIV positive employees being fired from their jobs, losing their health insurance benefits and their apartment lease, or of work colleagues moving the desk of a person known to be HIV positive to the other end of a room or demanding separate toilet or lunchroom or work facilities. For a person who has learned of his or her HIV seropositivity, that kind of social and economic ostracism can be deeply hurtful psychologically.

Of specific concern to chemical dependency treatment services is that such emotional cataclysm might cause a patient to relapse or leave treatment. Consider what it did to Patricia whose story was cited earlier in this chapter — a glaring example of what can happen under the influence of a mind-altering chemical like alcohol.

Testing with Counseling

The psychological pressures that play upon persons who are told they are HIV positive can be varied and unpredictable. Though most people respond to an HIV positive result by changing their lifestyle and taking action to protect others from infection, there are also those who react destructively, become suicidal, lose hope, and become vengeful to others. They seek to retaliate against those that they think infected them, or against a society that "allowed" the AIDS epidemic to happen. Because one of the widely held myths of AIDS is that HIV positivity equals infection equals AIDS equals death, there is understandably a good deal of panic tied in to a positive test result.

Most HIV positive patients ultimately approach the news with a sense of acceptance and determination to get their lives in order, write their wills, and take charge of their affairs.

Some feel frustration, anger, and lack of control over their future. Very few react with a desire to go out in a blaze of glory and damn the consequences — especially to others.

Even the most effective counseling can't anticipate all of the reactions possible in the face of an HIV positive result, and it won't mediate or deflect all of the frustration, anger, fear, and panic that might ensue. But it can help. And it can also have an educational effect on those who don't test positive, but were concerned enough about the possibility to have undergone the stress and risk of testing anyway.

Just as there are some people testing positive who might take a "damn the consequences" attitude, there are those with an HIV negative test who need a note of cautionary restraint. This point — not becoming overconfident in the face of a negative test — should be emphasized in counseling. The ELISA test detects antibodies to HIV. Because antibodies don't become detectable in all people at the same rate, a negative ELISA test does not necessarily mean the person tested is not infected. It could just mean that his or her infection is not yet detectable.

Seroconversion varies in individuals. Most people seroconvert — go from negative to positive — four to six weeks after exposure to HIV. But there are some who take a lot longer.[4] Rarely are people viremic but not seropositive.

There are studies indicating that some people may remain seronegative for over a year and then convert to positive. There are also reports that some individuals can test seropositive, revert to seronegative, and reconvert again to seropositive.

Thus there are people with an HIV negative test reading who are actually infectious for HIV and don't know it. If they use that "clean bill" to go back to a life of high-risk behavior, they may infect a lot of people before the hard truth of their HIV status is known.

Since the AIDS virus is not easily transmitted and is passed on only by the semen or blood of one person getting into another person, risk reduction is not difficult. That much has been learned of the AIDS epidemic. Even those who have been concerned enough about their own risk of infection to have taken the test — and have tested negative — should be counseled on the need for reducing high-risk behavior. They need to know that a negative test is no guarantee they are free of the HIV virus. Elimination of high-risk behavior is the best guarantee. They need to know that the HIV antibody test has shortcomings. And just as a positive HIV test does not mean a death sentence, a negative one does not mean immunity.

Mandatory Testing Versus Voluntary Testing

Since there are clear benefits as well as risks to HIV testing, the questions about testing usually boil down to, when and under what conditions should testing be mandatory? Or, should it ever be mandatory?

As AIDS has grown into a political issue, public figures have advocated many recommendations concerning testing: that all hospital patients be routinely tested for HIV upon admission, all couples applying for marriage licenses be tested, all patients in chemical dependency centers be tested, and all people applying for health insurance or being put into jails or joining the military be tested.

So far, mandatory testing of recruits into the military service and applicants for certain U.S. government service jobs and immigrants has been implemented. In some cases, a positive result leads to dismissal from a particular service. It may also mean restrictions on the kind of work an individual is allowed to do. Obviously, such widespread testing applied to the entire population of the U.S. would not only be extremely expensive, it would also raise some monumental problems, such as what do we do with the results? What do we do with hospital patients who are found HIV positive? Do we deny them admission? And if we admit them, do we treat them differently from other patients? And if we test all of these and other groups mandatorily, where do we get the resources, the money, the people, to provide the pre- and post-test counseling essential to any testing effort?

Voluntary testing is another matter. It has been argued that persons at risk for infection should be given every opportunity and encouragement for testing so long as that testing is supported by appropriate counseling, clear consent procedures, and strict confidentiality guarantees.

Most test sites say they maintain confidentiality. But the truth is that medical records, even ones reporting on HIV status, are often quite available to a large number of people, including not only hospital staff, but insurers, HMOs, employers, utilization and peer reviewers — the legions of people who make it their business to monitor the costs of patient care.

Thus, persons undergoing tests should know that claims of confidentiality, so routinely made by health care institutions, should not be taken for granted. People should also be told that in some locations, whether there is an assurance of confidentiality or not, HIV test results must be reported to certain public health authorities, and some of these have the power to isolate persons who test positive.

Anonymous Testing

Fear about misuse of test result information has spawned growth of many anonymous testing sites across the nation where numbers rather than names are used. Even at such sites, however, the need for counseling is paramount.

The use of anonymous testing has certainly added a layer of security to the confidentiality process. But some advocates of strong public health control measures frown on the use of anonymous test sites. They say public health authorities should know who these "carriers" are, and their sexual contacts should be traced back as far as possible. In several states, California among them, there is political action to ban anonymous testing and to require those who do the testing to report all positive HIV results to health officials.

Some states are also enacting a variety of laws regulating AIDS testing and insurance guidelines.

In the debate about mandatory versus voluntary testing, the point also has to be made that voluntary isn't always voluntary. There are many ways to encourage an individual to volunteer for a certain action or duty. Until such risks are addressed and such loopholes are plugged, even voluntary testing can be a risky undertaking. In the quest to expand HIV testing, there have been some wild expectations and rationalizations. But there have also been some thoughtful, reasoned justifications to use testing information in a positive way for public health purposes.

Testing is not a black and white issue with conservatives uniformly for it and liberals and civil rights advocates against it. The issue of testing is complex, and each decision to test or not to test should be made on an individual basis, with thoughtful consideration about the benefits and risks of testing for the person considering the test and for the society in which that person lives.

ENDNOTES

1. K. B. Meyer and S. G. Pauer, "Screening for HIV: Can We Afford the False Positive Rate?" *New England Journal of Medicine* vol. 317, no. 4 (23 July 1987): 238.

2. C. R. Schuster, "NIAAA/NADA Research on Alcohol and Drug Abuse and AIDS — Current Projects and Future Needs," in *Keeping Hope Alive,* Milan Korcok, ed. (Providence, Rhode Island: Manisses Communications, 1988), 47.

3. S. C. Joseph, "Current and Future Trends in AIDS in New York City," *Advances in Alcohol and Substance Abuse* vol. 7, no. 2 (1987): 159.

4. S. Nichols, "HIV Testing, Confidentiality and Anti-Discrimination Issues," in *Keeping Hope Alive*, Milan Korcok, ed. (Providence, Rhode Island: Manisses Communications, 1988), 44.

Liability and Confidentiality Issues

Fear in the CD Unit

With litigation as prevalent as it is, health care providers need to thoughtfully assess the risks of admitting or denying an AIDS or HIV positive patient to treatment. Some treatment centers see value in testing all incoming patients for HIV to keep those who test positive out of their program. They would rather others took in these patients.

They fear:

- HIV transmission to staff and other patients,
- the stigma of becoming known as a center that treats AIDS patients,
- that the demands of AIDS patients might upset their normal treatment process, and
- what such publicity might do to their business, their patient recruitment efforts, and their standing in the community.

Though many of these fears are rooted in ignorance of how difficult it really is for the AIDS virus to enter another person's body, they are genuine. And they can be dealt with only by credible, repeated, and persuasive education.

AIDS: The Drug and Alcohol Connection

Denying Treatment Is Discriminatory

Despite these fears, denying available and appropriate chemical dependency treatment to AIDS or HIV positive patiens is clearly discriminatory and contravenes the patient's rights. It is also bad for the public health as seropositive patients are far less likely to infect others if they are in treatment. In treatment HIV positive patients also appear to have a better prognosis, they stay healthier, and they retain a better quality of life.[1]

The Presidential Commission on the Human Immunodeficiency Virus Epidemic concluded that discrimination was the foremost obstacle to progress in fighting AIDS, and it recommended that federal legislation protect the rights to treatment of persons infected with HIV. The Commission also urged a massive expansion of the existing chemical dependency treatment system to allow any drug users who need and want treatment to get it.

The full report of the presidential commission is available in most libraries. Its recommendations are far-reaching and focus tightly on the connection between drug use and AIDS.

The medical profession has also come out strongly in favor of fighting discrimination towards AIDS and HIV positive patients.

The American Medical Association Council on Ethical and Judicial Affairs' policy on treating patients with HIV disease is clear: "A physician may not ethically refuse to treat a patient whose condition is within the physician's current realm of competence solely because the patient is HIV-antibody positive."

And a ". . . physician . . . unable to provide services should make referrals to those physicians or facilities equipped to do so." These and other recommendations about HIV testing are available in *HIV Blood Testing Counseling: AMA Physician Guidelines*, published by the Division of Health Science, American

Medical Association, 535 North Dearborn St., Chicago, IL 60610.

The American College of Physicians, headquartered in Philadelphia, also has approved a policy saying that refusal of a physician to care for a specific category of patients — for example, patients who have AIDS or are HIV positive — "is morally and ethically indefensible."

The American Medical Society on Alcoholism and Other Drug Dependencies (AMSAODD), headquartered in New York City and which represents physicians specializing in the addictions, says that physicians, other health professionals, and programs for the treatment of alcoholism and other drug dependencies should provide treatment for HIV positive patients. It says further that patients with AIDS do not require infection control techniques different from patients with hepatitis B. AMSAODD's position on such treatment has been published in its *Guidelines For Facilities Treating Chemically Dependent Patients at Risk for AIDS or Infected by HIV Virus.*

As policies and laws to prevent discrimination against AIDS and HIV positive patients become more commonplace, the legal risks of denying such patients a place in chemical dependency treatment will grow increasingly hazardous.

Precautions Are Necessary

But at the same time, there's no absence of risk in admitting AIDS and HIV positive patients into treatment. Precautions need to be taken for the sake of staff, other patients, and the families and friends of HIV positive patients.

Voluntary testing of patients at high risk for HIV infection can offer useful information for their own treatment, and is encouraged by many chemical dependency professionals so long as it is accompanied by appropriate pre- and post-test counseling and adequate confidentiality measures.

Using Test Information

But testing raises dilemmas and questions, as we discussed in the previous chapter. If a therapist yields to a patient's refusal to tell others in the group that he or she is HIV positive and another patient or staff member subsequently becomes infected, might the therapist and the facility itself not be sued by the newly infected person? On the other hand, if the therapist uses privileged information to warn other patients about an HIV positive person in their midst, is he or she not contravening a person's right to confidentiality?

The American Medical Society on Alcoholism and Other Drug Dependencies, in its guidelines referred to earlier, suggest that because the incubation period of HIV can last for years, it would be very difficult to pinpoint exactly when infection occurred, or even that a person was infectious at the time he or she was in the program. Nonetheless, legal actions have been taken on less expensive affairs (and once taken, legal proceedings can be torturous).

While health care professionals have a responsibility to protect the confidentiality of their patient's medical records, they also have other patients and the public health to consider. Although the risk of a patient becoming infected by HIV is no greater in a properly run chemical dependency center than it is in a hotel or a theater, the sensitivities of other patients and the aims of the treatment program can't be ignored. Most group sessions are based on openness and probity and sharing of deeply personal thoughts and feelings. Participants are urged and encouraged to tell the truth about themselves and discuss their fears and anxieties.

How can the professional facilitators of such sessions maintain their honesty and integrity if they cover up for a patient with AIDS? How can others in the group keep from feeling betrayed when and if they find out about the cover-up?

And how can a patient who is already vulnerable be expected to handle the possible rejection and ostracism of others in his or her group should the truth of HIV or AIDS status be revealed?

Confidentiality Versus the Public Health

Physicians and other health care workers have an obligation to (1) protect patients' confidentiality, and (2) preserve the public health. Occasionally, these obligations collide, leaving the professional with an agonizing choice.

If an AIDS or HIV positive patient avoids telling a partner that he or she is at risk for infection, and that patient continues unsafe behaviors, how does the caregiver warn the partner without contravening the patient's confidentiality? And is the caregiver legally liable for having broken the confidence? On the other hand, is the caregiver not legally liable if he or she does not take steps to protect family or the public health? These are tough questions the courts and medical ethicists are just beginning to deal with.

Some states require all doctors to report positive tests to the state health department.

In New York State, the law now gives doctors immunity from legal action by their AIDS or HIV positive patients if they inform their patients' sexual or intravenous drug using partners of the HIV risk.

The American Medical Association's policy (as outlined in the HIV testing publication cited earlier in this chapter) recommends that doctors warn sex partners of AIDS virus carriers of their risk if their patients or other state authorities fail to do so. But the policy also says physicians should breach the confidentiality of their patients only as a last resort necessary to protect unsuspecting people.

What to do about medical records containing HIV information is still another question. Withholding laboratory results from a patient's chart is illegal and unethical. Some hospitals are now separating out information about HIV status and allowing its release only with the consent of the patient.

The protection of confidentiality is a matter chemical dependency professionals deal with every day. The advent of HIV Spectrum Disease into the chemical dependency treatment system will clearly heighten the need to become even more rigorous about that protection.

ENDNOTES

1. D. Smith, "Integrating AIDS Education and Treatment With Chemical Dependency Treatment," in *Keeping Hope Alive*, Milan Korcok, ed. (Providence, Rhode Island: Manisses Communications, 1988), 63.

CHAPTER ELEVEN

Recovery from AIDS and Addiction

The goal of this book has been to demystify AIDS, to Keep It Simple, to provide information clearly, and to differentiate perceptions from realities. One of the realities about AIDS is that recovery is possible.

Much of medicine, and all of the popular media, has tended to equate AIDS with a death sentence. And very often when you tell somebody they are going to die, they do. It's amazing how far some people will go to please their doctors!

Some Patients Beat the Odds

On the other hand, there are numerous examples of people beating the odds: cancer patients with unexplainable spontaneous remissions, individuals in prolonged comas who miraculously wake up, and AIDS patients who recover.

Case History

Ron was the most popular doctor on the hospital staff. When he developed Kaposi's sarcoma, everyone was upset. Chemotherapy didn't help, and he rapidly became unable to continue his hospital work. Then he developed pneumonia and was hospitalized.

One complication followed another. He was moved to the intensive care unit where his kidneys failed, requiring artificial kidney treatment. Then, liver failure occurred and his blood pressure became impossible to maintain, even with drugs.

A deep coma ensued and Ron became unresponsive; only a breathing machine maintained his blood oxygen level, and only a tiny blip on the heart monitor and another blip showing a very slight brain wave indicated any evidence of life.

As his doctor and friend, I, Dr. Larry Siegel, came to his bedside very early one morning, about 3 A.M. I shed my tears and wrote the final "Do Not Resuscitate" orders that he arranged for in his will. I said my farewell, wishing him a safe journey. All medical miracles had failed. There was nothing else to do. I let go. Very sadly, very reluctantly, I let go.

About noon, the intensive care unit nurses called and said Ron's blood pressure was holding a little better with less medicine. Three days later his kidneys began to work and soon the breathing machine was removed.

A month later, Ron walked out of the hospital.

He said to me later, "I saw you all standing there. I was up above you, and there was a great feeling of peace. But I knew there were some things I had to do."

Ron lived to take care of much "unfinished business" with many people in his life. I saw him riding his bike a few months later, absolutely joyously.

Such recovery is, of course, a rare event. But life is made up of events, common and rare. That's why the words "never" or "always" should be used with reservation.

Many who became ill with the plague in the Middle Ages, or who contracted polio or influenza in the earlier part of this century, recovered completely from what were then known as "fatal" or "nearly always fatal" diseases. Most of those people recovered without the benefit of space age technology.

And what about the millions who have recovered from the "seemingly hopeless state of mind and body" — the disease of alcoholism? So it is with AIDS. There are survivors. There are people with full-blown Centers for Disease Control AIDS who are well, alive, and functioning five, six, seven or more years after their diagnosis.

84

Case History

In 1983, Michael had cryptosporidiosis, a debilitating AIDS re-
lated intestinal parasite. Since then he has had a variety of bacterial
and fungal infections. He refuses to take any of the standard treat-
ments for HIV diseases except pentamidine, a preventive medication
for AIDS-related Pneumocystis Carinii pneumonia.

Michael describes himself as an agnostic or atheist, not at all
spiritual. He drinks cola all the time, but uses no other mood-altering
drugs.

Michael spends his days telling all who will listen that survival
from AIDS is possible. "Just go for it!" he says. He has helped
innumerable people with HIV disease through his extensive writings,
talks, and music. He is deeply commited to his lover, who is also
deeply commited to him. His somewhat sarcastic sense of humor is
infectious and he clearly loves life.

Michael is a long-term survivor, and despite his declaration of
agnosticism or atheism, he is one of the most spiritual people I have
ever met.

If one uses Centers for Disease Control data, even taking
into account the agency's decision to reclassify people with
PCP, Kaposi's sarcoma, and other AIDS diagnoses as not
having AIDS if they are alive and HIV seronegative, it's clear
that some people who have had AIDS since 1981 are still alive.

A study published in the *New England Journal of Medicine*
evaluated the probability of five year survival with AIDS,
based on data from 5,800 people with AIDS. It showed that
the probability for five year survival is 15 percent for all persons with AIDS, and up to 30 percent for gay men with
Kaposi's sarcoma.[1]

There are also a few documented cases of individuals who
have become infected, developed typical antibody responses
— which were verified — and then went on to clear their
bodies with no evidence of subsequent infection.[2]

While most of these people have been shown to have a

residual viral "footprint," there is at least one formerly infected person who doesn't show even this evidence of residual infection.[3]

Certainly, there will be more, longer term survivors as our technology improves, as our methods of diagnosis and treatment become more sophisticated, as new drugs to fight AIDS and its manifestations are developed, as we begin to treat HIV positive people at earlier stages in their disease, and as we become more aggressive in implementing approved and even unapproved but clinically effective therapeutic regimens.

Empowering Patients

One of the most effective of these regimens is the support of empowerment for clients and patients.

As caregivers work through the stages of grief and loss when a person discovers he or she is positive for HIV, we can offer information, we can counsel him or her about behavioral risks, and we can provide hope. Caregivers can enter into a partnership, a therapeutic alliance with the patient.

Caregivers can listen and learn from patients, as patients can learn from caregivers. This is the essence of empowerment. This is the willingness to have a partnership. For physicians, to become an attending physician means to pay attention.

What happens to empowered patients with AIDS? And why? First of all, some survive. All of the long-term survivors have what one observer calls "grit." In *Love, Medicine and Miracles*, a book by Dr. Bernie Siegel, numerous examples of patients beating their disease are cited. Some of the characteristics of these winners are that they have complex biphasic traits: they are both serious and playful, tough and gentle, logical and intuitive, hard-working and lazy. They are also aggressive, flexible, adaptive, and have highly developed self-esteem and intelligence. They are not docile.

Case History

Joey was the best worker in the plant. Never sick, never missed a day. Everyone at work knew that Chip and he had been lovers for five years. Still, he played on the plant's baseball team and occasionally had a few beers after work with co-workers — "a real, regular guy."

When his headaches became blinding, he could no longer ignore them and the plant nurse immediately referred him to a physician. A CAT scan of his brain showed a solitary lesion with a bright ring around it, typical for toxoplasmosis. The chest x-ray showed typical pneumocystis carinii pneumonia. Chip freaked out and left town.

Joey got mad! He decided that no damn disease was going to get him without a good fight. He started to read books about survivors. He read Siegel's Love, Medicine & Miracles, and Louise Hay's The AIDS Book — Creating a Positive Approach. He joined a therapy group and stopped using all alcohol and other drugs, including his favorite "poppers" he used during sex or at the disco.

The medications for his opportunistic infections worked and he began to feel well again. He began a program of medical therapy including vitamins, zidovudine (formerly known as AZT), and Fansidar (to prevent recurrent toxoplasmosis and pneumocystis pneumonia).

He exercised regularly for the first time in years, stopped smoking, and ate a very healthy diet. He gained weight and energy. He took charge, learned all about his illness, refused to take any medications unless they were thoroughly explained and made sense to him, and refused any rooms in hospitals, when necessary, unless they had a view of the water.

He was a little irritating to all the health care workers involved with him, but they admired his grit.

Today, three years later, Joey continues to work full time and looks and feels well, though he is still on medication. He is very clear in stating what he wants and usually gets it. He loves life and is open to a relationship with someone he started dating.

The Influence of the Brain on Disease

As alluded to briefly in Chapter Four, psychoneuroimmunology is an emerging field of medicine that is particularly relevant to the treatment and management of AIDS. It is concerned with the interactions between the central nervous system and the immune system. It originated in the 1960s with the hypothesis that stress can suppress the immune system, and has expanded from there to probe the many influences the emotions can have on the course of disease.

Anatomic and biochemical connections between the brain and the immune system are known to exist. We have seen that it is possible to enhance T-cell numbers and function with chemicals that mimic or increase naturally occurring neuropeptides produced in the parts of the brain concerned with emotions. Examples are met-enkephlin, imreg, and naltrexone.

Other neuropeptides, such as "Peptide T," modulated by the central nervous system, may directly block the attachment of HIV to the T-4 receptor sites, thus preventing damage. The depletion of these same neurotransmitter groups in chemically dependent individuals, and their return to normal during recovery from addiction, has received considerable experimental attention and support. The enhancement of T-cells by exercise, perhaps mediated by endorphins or other neurotransmitters, has also recently been demonstrated.

A discussion of neuropeptides can easily lapse into the esoteric for those whose prime concern is dealing with the day-to-day sensitivities and emergencies of AIDS and HIV positive patients in the chemical dependency setting. But the need to link what goes on in the brain and how it affects the immune and other body systems is fundamental for professionals in chemical dependency settings.

The Unique Role of CD Caregivers

Whether by deliberate action or by circumstance, these chemical dependency caregivers will find themselves on the front line in the fight against AIDS. No one is better equipped to meet this challenge. No one knows better the devastating effects of alcohol and other drugs on the mind, body, and spirit. No one knows better how to diagnose the use and abuse of mood-, mind-, and body-altering chemicals. No one is more adept at dealing with the denial, stigma, and shame that encompasses alcoholics, other drug addicts, and people with AIDS. No one is more skilled in enlisting family, lovers, friends, employers, and other health professionals to participate in the process of intervention, Twelve Step recovery, and relapse prevention.

The same recovery-oriented, abstinence-based treatment that allows people to recover from alcoholism and other addictions, may also help AIDS patients recover from AIDS, and enhance the chance of survival or quality of life of those who are HIV positive. The help offered by the professional recovery community is a rare comfort at a time when effective medications are few, the process to develop them is slow, and the proposition that things will get worse before they get better seems a certainty.

ENDNOTES

1. R. Rothenberg, et al., "Survival With the Acquired Immunodeficiency Syndrome," *New England Journal of Medicine*, vol. 317, no. 21 (19 November 1897): 1,297.
2. H. Burger et al., "Transient Antibody to Lymphadenopathy Associated Virus/HTLV III and T-Lymphocyte Abnormalities in the Wife of a Man who Developed Acquired Immune Deficiency Disease," *Annals of Internal Medicine*, vol. 103, no. 4 (October 1985): 545.

3. H. Farzadegan et al., "Loss Of Human Immunodeficiency Virus Type I (HIV-I) Antibodies with Evidence of Viral Infection In Asymptomatic Homosexual Men," *Annals of Internal Medicine,* vol. 108, no. 6 (June 1985): 785.

Centers for Disease Control Universal Precautions

These Universal Blood and Body Fluid Precautions were excerpted from the Centers for Disease Control Morbidity and Mortality Weekly Report 1987, *Volume 36, Number 2S and Centers for Disease Control* Morbidity and Mortality Weekly Report 1988 *Volume 37, Number 24.*

Since medical history and examination cannot reliably identify all patients infected with HIV or other blood-borne pathogens, blood and body-fluid precautions should be used consistently for all patients. This approach, previously recommended by CDC, and referred to as "universal blood and body-fluid precautions" or "universal precautions," should be used in the care of all patients, especially including those in emergency-care settings in which the risk of blood exposure is increased and the infection status of the patient is usually unknown.

1. All healthcare workers should routinely use appropriate barrier precautions to prevent skin and mucous-membrane exposure when contact with blood or other body fluids such as vomitus, urine, or fecal matter which contains visible blood of any patient is anticipated. Gloves should be worn for touching blood and body fluids in which one can see blood, mucous membranes, or non-intact skin of all patients, for handling items or surfaces soiled with blood or body fluids, and for performing venipuncture and other vascular access proce-

dures. Gloves should be changed after contact with each patient. Masks and protective eyewear or face shields should be worn during procedures that are likely to generate droplets of blood or other blood-containing body fluids to prevent exposure of mucous membranes of the mouth, nose, and eyes. Gowns or aprons should be worn during procedures that are likely to generate splashes of blood or other visible blood-containing body fluids.

2. Hands and other skin surfaces should be washed immediately and thoroughly if contaminated with blood or other body fluids. Hands should be washed immediately after gloves are removed.

3. All health-care workers should take precautions to prevent injuries caused by needles, scalpels, and other sharp instruments or devices during procedures; when cleaning used instruments; during disposal of used needles; and when handling sharp instruments after procedures. To prevent needlestick injuries, needles should not be recapped, purposely bent or broken by hand, removed from disposable syringes, or otherwise manipulated by hand. After they are used, disposable syringes and needles, scalpel blades, and other sharp items should be placed in puncture-resistant containers for disposal; the puncture-resistant containers should be located as close as practical to the use area. Large-bore reusable needles should be placed in a puncture-resistant container for transport to the reprocessing area.

4. Although saliva has not been implicated in HIV transmission, to minimize the need for emergency mouth-to-mouth resuscitation, mouthpieces, resuscitation bags, or other ventilation devices should be available for use in areas in which the need for resuscitation is predictable.

5. Health-care workers who have exudative lesions or weeping dermatitis should refrain from all direct patient care and from handling patient-care equipment until the condition resolves.

6. Pregnant health-care workers are not known to be at

greater risk of contracting HIV infection than health-care workers who are not pregnant; however, if a health-care worker develops HIV infection during pregnancy, the infant is at risk of infection resulting from perinatal transmission. Because of this risk, pregnant health-care workers should be especially familiar with and strictly adhere to precautions to minimize the risk of HIV transmission.

Implementation of universal blood and body-fluid precautions for *all* patients eliminates the need for use of the isolation category of "Blood and Body Fluid Precautions" previously recommended by CDC for patients known or suspected to be infected with blood-borne pathogens. Isolation precautions (e.g., enteric, AFB) should be used as necessary if associated conditions, such as infectious diarrhea or tuberculosis, are diagnosed or suspected.

Precautions for Invasive Procedures

In this document, an invasive procedure is defined as surgical entry into tissues, cavities, or organs or repair of major traumatic injuries 1) in an operating or delivery room, emergency department, or outpatient setting, including both physicians' and dentists' offices; 2) cardiac catheterization and angiographic procedures; 3) a vaginal or cesarean delivery or other invasive obstetric procedure during which bleeding may occur; or 4) the manipulation, cutting, or removal of any oral or perioral tissues, including tooth structure, during which bleeding occurs or the potential for bleeding exists. The universal blood and body-fluid precautions listed above, combined with the precautions listed below, should be the minimum precautions for *all* such invasive procedures.

1. All health-care workers who participate in invasive procedures must routinely use appropriate barrier precautions to prevent skin and mucous-membrane contact with blood and other body fluids of all patients. Gloves and surgical masks must be worn for all invasive procedures. Protective eyewear

or face shields should be worn for procedures that commonly result in the generation of droplets, splashing of blood or other body fluids, or the generation of bone chips. Gowns or aprons made of materials that provide an effective barrier should be worn during invasive procedures that are likely to result in the splashing of blood or other body fluids. All health-care workers who perform or assist in vaginal or cesarean deliveries should wear gloves and gowns when handling the placenta or the infant until blood and amniotic fluid have been removed from the infant's skin and should wear gloves during post-delivery care of the umbilical cord.

2. If a glove is torn or a needlestick or other injury occurs, the glove should be removed and a new glove used as promptly as patient safety permits; the needle or instrument involved in the incident should also be removed from the sterile field.

Condom Use

Buying and using a condom should not be a forbidding or embarrassing experience. What follows are points for clinical staff to ask when discussing the use of condoms with patients.

When to Buy Condoms

Not at three o'clock in the morning when the urge arrives but the drugstores are all closed. Plan ahead.

Buy a reasonable supply. Don't plan on keeping them for a long time. Carrying them in one's wallet or purse for long periods affects their reliability. Condoms have a shelf life. Check the expiration date on the package. Don't buy old ones.

The most reliable are made of latex. Don't buy them if they are made of any other materials. Also, they should have a reservoir (nipple) end, and they should be lubricated with a substance containing nonoxynol 9, which helps prevent against sexually transmitted diseases.

If the condom is unlubricated, don't use oil-based substances like vasoline. Use only water-soluble lubricants or spermicidal jellies.

Store condoms in a cool, dry place — not in a glove compartment. Heat can deteriorate them.

Carry one at all times.

How to Put a Condom On

Don't remove the condom from its package until it's time to put it on. Then, carefully roll it down over the penis to the base. Do this before you start foreplay. Don't wait until you're ready to penetrate, that's risky. Drops of semen may already have started oozing.

Leave some space at the tip to catch the semen.

Taking the Condom Off

Hold the condom at the base of the penis and withdraw soon after ejaculation. You don't want the condom to come off a soft penis that is still inside your partner.

Take it off carefully, keep the condom and its contents away from your partner, and dispose of it safely. Immediately wash away any semen that may have spilled, and do not allow semen to come into contact with cuts or breaks in the skin.

Never reuse a condom.

Suggested Reading

Books

"Acquired Immunodeficiency Syndrome: Position paper of the Health and Public Policy Committee, American College of Physicians, and the Infectious Diseases Society of America," *Annals of Internal Medicine*, vol. 104, no. 4 (April 1986): 575.

AIDS and Substance Abuse. Larry Siegel, M.D., ed. New York: Hayworth Press, 1988.

Fortunato, John E. *AIDS: The Spiritual Dilemma.* San Francisco: Harper and Row, 1987.

Hay, Louise, L. *AIDS: A Positive Approach.* Santa Monica, Calif.: Hay House, 1988. (audiocassette)

Hay, Louise, L. *The AIDS Book — Creating a Positive Approach.* Santa Monica, Calif.: Hay House, 1988.

Selwyn, P. *AIDS: What Is Now Known.* New York: HPB Publishing, 1986.

Siegel, Bernie S. *Love, Medicine, and Miracles.* San Francisco: Harper and Row, 1987.

Siegel, Larry, M.D. *AIDS, Alcohol and Drugs — The Video.* Naples, Fla.: Health Care Network, Inc., 1988. (videotape)

Tilleraas, Perry. *The Color of Light: Daily Meditations for All of Us Living with AIDS.* Center City, Minn.: Hazelden Educational Materials, 1988.

Articles

"Acquired Immune Deficiency and Chemical Dependency"
Symposium Proceedings NCA/AMSAODD Meeting, April 1986
Department of Health and Human Services Publication No. (ADM) 87-1513
U.S. Department of Health and Human Services
Public Health Service

Alcohol, Drug Abuse and Mental Health Administration
NIAAA
5600 Fishers Lane
Rockville, MD 20857

"AIDS: Perceptions vs. Realities."
Journal of Psychoactive Drugs, vol. 20 (1988): 149-52.
Larry Siegel, M.D.
520 Southard Street
Key West, FL 33040

"AIDS: Relationship to Alcohol and Other Drugs."
Journal of Substance Abuse Treatment, vol. 3 (1986): 271-74
Larry Siegel, M.D.
520 Southard Street
Key West, FL 33040

Guidelines for Facilities Treating Chemically Dependent Patients at Risk for AIDS or Infected by HIV Virus, 2nd ed.,1988.
Distributed for AMSAODD by:
PROHEALTH
P.O. Box 11180
Ft. Lauderdale , FL 33339
(305) 561-5352

Keeping Hope Alive
Proceedings of the Second National Forum on AIDS and Chemical Dependency, 1988
Manisses Publications
3 Governor Square
P.O. Box 3357 Wayland Square
Providence, RI 02906-0357

Surgeon General's Report on AIDS
U.S. Public Health Service
Public Affairs Office
Hubert H. Humphrey Building #725 H
200 Independence Avenue S.W.
Washington DC 20201
(202) 245-6867

INDEX

A

Acquired Immune Deficiency Syndrome, 1-4, 7-9, 14; among women, 12; and condom use, 56, 61, 95-96; and treatment of chemically dependent patients, 43-48; average time from infection to, 14; cofactors, 10-11; diagnosing, 47-48; education, 34-39, 45-47; high-risk behaviors, 18, 27-28, 55-59; in children, 18-20; prevention of, 34, 45-46; recovery from, 83-89; seropositivity among IV drug users, 4, 43, 68; survival, 14, 21-22, 85; symptoms of, 47. *See also* Human Immunodeficiency Virus Infection

AIDS. *See* Acquired Immune Deficiency Syndrome

AIDS dementia, 48

AIDS Related Conditions, 13

Alcohol: disinhibition by, 7-28; use of, and immune function, 26-27

American College of Physicians, 78

American Medical Association, 78, 81

American Medical Society on Alcoholism and Other Drug Dependencies, 3, 79, 80

Amnesic spells, 47

AMSAODD. *See* American Medical Society on Alcoholism and Other Drug Dependencies

Anal intercourse. *See* Rectal intercourse

Anonymous testing, 74-75

Aphasia, 47

ARC. *See* AIDS Related Conditions

Autologous blood, 21

Azidothymidine, 33, 70

AZT. *See* Azidothymidine

B

Basophils, 8

Benzodiazepines, 26

Drug use: and immune function, 26-27, 60; disinhibition, 27-28; use of unsterile injection equipment, 17-18

E
ELISA. *See* Enzyme-Linked Immunosorbent Assay
Enzyme-Linked Immunosorbent Assay, use and limitations of, 10, 63-64
Eosinophils, 8
Ethical guidelines and policies on AIDS, 78-79
Ethyl chloride, 28

F
Families, importance of AIDS education to, 37-39
Fear: among health care professionals, 34, 45, 77; dealing with, 34-37
Fever, 13

G
Gay community: chemical abuse in, 29; AIDS survival, 22
Global loss of affect, 47
Grief, dealing with, 39-40
Guided imagery, 31, 34

H
HIV. *See* Human Immunodeficiency Virus
HIV Infection. *See* Human Immunodeficiency Virus Infection
HIV Spectrum Disease, 13
HIV Testing: anonymous testing, 74-75; benefits of, 69-70; consent form, 67-68; ELISA, 10, 63-64; guidelines on, 66-67; IFA, 64; importance of counseling, 71-73; limitations of, 10, 65; mandatory and voluntary testing, 73-74; need for confidentiality, 64; risks of, 71; Western Blot, 10, 64
Health care professionals: and counseling, 33, 52, 56-58; determining high-risk behaviors, 55-56; diagnosing

AIDS, 47-48; ethical guidelines, 77-79; fear among, 34,
45, 77; importance of attitude, 44-45; making referrals,
40; HIV exposure and seroconversion among, 12, 50-51;
need for AIDS education, 34
Helper cells, 8
Heroin, 26
Heterosexual contact, 12
High-risk behaviors, 18, 27-28, 55-59
Human Immunodeficiency Virus, 7; and AIDS
development, 9; exposure to, in Americans, 13; means of
transmission, 12, 50, 55-56, 58-59
Human Immunodeficiency Virus Infection, 17; among IV
drug users, 4, 43, 68; and blood transfusions, 21;
improving immune status, 51-52; high-risk behaviors
and, 55-57; prevention, 34, 55-61; signs and symptoms
of, 13, 40, 46; undetected, 49-50

I
IFA. *See* Indirect Immunofluorescence Assay
Indirect Immunofluorescense Assay, 64
Immune system: enhancement of, 51-52, 88; suppression
of, 9, 60; understanding the, 25, 30-31
Intravenous drug use, and AIDS, 12, 18
Intravenous drug users, seropositivity among, 4, 43, 68

K
Kaposi's sarcoma, 13, 14, 22, 26
Koop, C. Everett, Surgeon General, 1

L
Legal issues, 77-80
Liability issues, 77-80
Lymphocytes, 8

M
Macrophages, 8, 25
Mandatory HIV testing, 73
Marijuana, 26, 28
Media, impact of, 46
Meditation, 31
Memory loss, 47
Mirror work, 31, 34
Monocytes, 8
Morbidity and Mortality Weekly Report, 31
Mucous membrane linings, 7

N
National Institute of Child Health and Human
   Development, 19
Natural killer cells, 25-26
Needle-sharing, 17, 18, 58-59
Negative behavior, and body's immune system, 30-31
Neurocognitive defects, 13
Nitrites, 26, 28
N-K cells. *See* Natural killer cells
Nonoxynol 9, 56, 57-58, 61
Nutrition, importance of, 51-52

O
Opiates, 26
Opportunistic infections, 8
Oral contraceptives, 26
Outreach programs, 59-61

P
Plasma, 8
Pneumococcal pneumonia, 13
Pneumocystis carinii pneumonia, 13
Polymorphenuclear leukocytes, 8
Poppers, 26, 28

U
Universal Blood and Body Fluid Precautions, 14, 45, 50, 61, 91-94
Universal Body Substance Isolation Precautions, 14
U.S. Department of Health and Human Services, 19

V
Vaginal intercourse, 17, 18, 58
Voluntary testing, 74, 75

W
White blood cells, 8
Weight loss, 13
Western Blot, 10, 64

Z
Zidovudine, 33, 70

Other titles that will interest you

The Color of Light
Daily Meditations for All of Us Living with AIDS
by Perry Tilleraas
Recovery and the Twelve Step life give us the most important keys for effectively responding to AIDS, including the practice of daily meditation. Of special interest to people with AIDS or ARC, and those close to them, these meditations examine the spectrum of issues surrounding AIDS with a unique blend of spiritual and temporal wisdom. 400 pp.
Order No. 5056

Ethics for Addiction Professionals
by LeClair Bissell, M.D., C.A.C.
and James E. Royce, S.J., Ph.D.
Crucial and complex ethical issues are facing professionals in the addiction field today. The authors point out the necessity of standard guidelines for professional conduct by raising several key questions concerning confidentiality, credentialing, AIDS, counselor relapse, economics, and more. 60 pp.
Order No. 5028

Dual Identities
Counseling Chemically Dependent Gay Men and Lesbians
by Dana Finnegan, Ph.D. and Emily McNally, M.Ed.
This sensitive guide shows how we can use familiar counseling techniques to deal with the special needs and issues of gay and lesbian alcoholics. 128 pp.
Order No. 5011
